MAXIMUS BODY

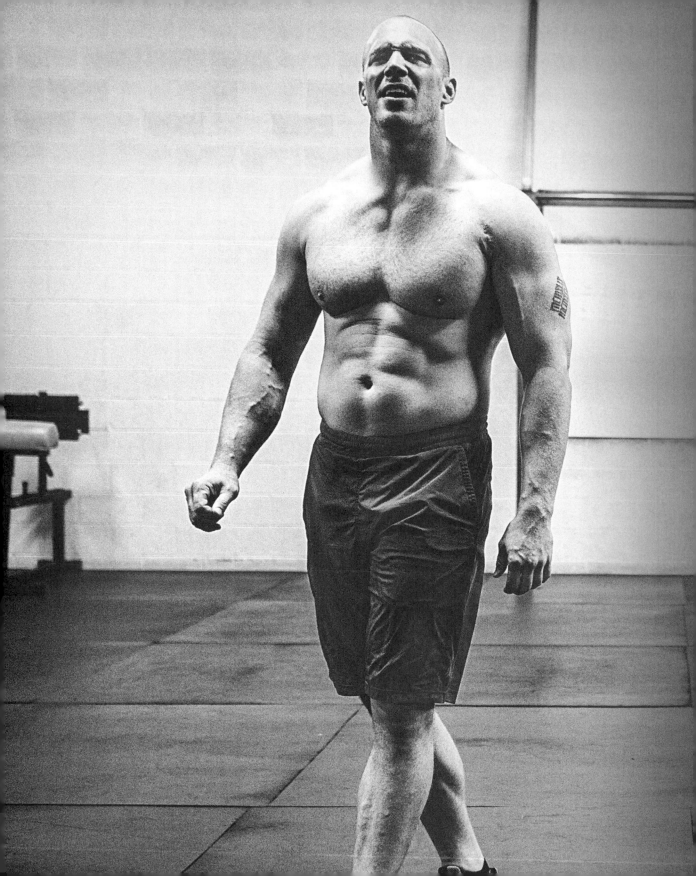

A Men'sHealth BOOK

THE PHYSICAL AND MENTAL TRAINING PLAN THAT SHREDS YOUR BODY, BUILDS SERIOUS STRENGTH, AND MAKES YOU UNSTOPPABLY FIT

MAXIMUS BODY

BOBBY MAXIMUS and MICHAEL EASTER

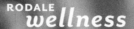

RODALE
wellness

Live happy. Be healthy. Get inspired.

Sign up today to get exclusive access to our authors, exclusive bonuses, and the most authoritative, useful, and cutting-edge information on health, wellness, fitness, and living your life to the fullest.

Visit us online at RodaleWellness.com
Join us at RodaleWellness.com/Join

First published in hardcover by Rodale Inc. in January 2017.
First published in paperback by Rodale Inc. in March 2018.

© 2017 by Rob MacDonald

Printed in the United States of America

Rodale Inc. makes every effort to use acid-free ∞, recycled paper ♻.

The photo credits appear on page 266.

Book design by Joanna Williams

Library of Congress Cataloging-in-Publication Data is on file with the publisher.

ISBN 978-1-62336-847-0   hardcover

ISBN 978-1-62336-990-3   paperback

Distributed to the trade by Macmillan

2   4   6   8   10   9   7   5   3   hardcover
2   4   6   8   10   9   7   5   3   1   paperback

 RODALE

Follow us @RodaleBooks on

We inspire health, healing, happiness, and love in the world.
Starting with you.

TO EVERYONE WHO WANTS TO MAKE
A BETTER LIFE FOR THEMSELVES. DREAMS CAN COME TRUE.
YOU JUST HAVE TO WORK HARD FOR THEM.

CONTENTS

SECTION I: PSYCHOLOGY

REAL FITNESS STARTS WITH WORKING THE MUSCLE INSIDE YOUR SKULL.

SECTION II: TRAINING

NOTHING WORTHWHILE WAS EVER EASY.

SECTION III: SUPPORT

TRAINING IS MORE THAN JUST THE TIME YOU SPEND IN THE GYM.

PART 1: NUTRITION 74

PART 2: RECOVERY 98

SECTION IV: THE MAXIMUS METHOD

BECOME THE FITTEST PERSON YOU KNOW.

SECTION V: THE MAXIMUS MANUAL

MORE THAN 100 OF THE BEST WORKOUTS YOU'LL EVER DO.

FOREWORD

I first heard of Bobby while reporting a story for *Men's Health* magazine, where I'm an editor. I'd sent out a mass e-mail to the best and brightest minds in the health and fitness industry, asking them a simple question: Who are some of the fittest men in the world?

Each source replied with a list of three or four names, most of whom were professional athletes. But the name that popped up most often in the replies was someone I'd never heard of: Bobby Maximus, a trainer.

This impossibly large Canadian, who is directly responsible for the success of a Salt Lake City-based gym called Gym Jones, they said, was not only breaking fitness records but also helping professional athletes win championships and transforming average guys into virtual superheroes.

A little research on the man and the gym where he works took me to a surprising Web site. Unlike most gym or trainer sites, no pop-ups greeted me with promises of six-pack abs in 4 weeks, limited-time offers for secret online coaching, or life-changing fitness information that I'd learn if I'd just sign up for their e-mail list. The Web site had no sales pitches. It centered on black-and-white photos of the most in-shape-looking people I'd ever seen, exercising far harder than I ever had. But beyond just abs and sweat, there was something else these people had, which rang through in each photo: an intangible air of confidence and competence.

The place and its head trainer, it seemed, were 100 percent real and free of gimmicks, something that often feels impossible to find in the fitness industry. I had to go there.

And so, half a decade ago, I stepped through the doors of Gym Jones to meet Bobby. After some general introductions, I asked him my typical health and fitness editor questions about what exercises he prefers, what training methods he thinks are best, and so on. He stopped me. "Exercises are always secondary to effort," he said. "And the latter is what most people struggle with—they do half-ass workouts, they make excuses, and they sell themselves short." That's why he's more concerned with first helping you get your mind right. "Have a strong mind," he said, and putting forth the effort becomes easy.

"Take you, for example," he continued. "What's your fitness goal, and how are you going to accomplish it?"

I mentioned a few goals I'd been working on for far too long, explaining that it can be tough to train enough because I work about 50 hours a week. He laughed and directed me to a big whiteboard on the wall of the Spartan gym's training room. Then he wrote "168" on the board and walked me through one of his infamous "time audits." (The number 168 is the number of hours in a week. You'll see how this factors in when you take your own time audit.) When it was over, I wanted to punch Dobby. I didn't, of course. Not just because he's an overwhelmingly large, ex-UFC fighter, but also because I knew he was right, and I was frustrated that he'd brought excuses to the surface that I didn't even realize I was telling myself.

Then he asked, "Ready to get to work?" I was, and over that weekend I learned many more hard truths; chief among them was that my definition of "my best" was nowhere close to my actual best. That weekend, filled with sweat and hard truths, changed the way I look at fitness forever.

Hard truths are like medicine: They don't always go down easy, but they're worth it because they make you better. So, I started taking Bobby's medicine regularly. Once I did that, everything changed. I became fitter than I had ever been, and I accomplished all of those goals that had once eluded me—and more. Through that, I adopted a no-excuse attitude that helps me with anything life throws my way.

As an editor of the world's biggest, most-influential health and fitness magazine, I've written thousands of articles about fitness. I've visited hundreds of gyms, talked to thousands of experts, tried a million different ways to train, and seen it all. And I can tell you this: No one else does what Bobby does. He does a better job transforming people—no matter how out-of-shape, hardheaded, or lost—than anyone in the country.

Follow Bobby's teachings, and it won't just be your body that becomes tougher; so will your mind. Once you have that, you'll cross some invisible line into a level of incredible fitness and tough-as-nails spirit that improves your entire life. Everything will come easier, whether it's picking up something heavy, accomplishing a big goal, or just dealing with the hardships of everyday life.

I wrote this book with Bobby because the health fitness industry is failing people. The pitch that getting healthy and fit is quick and easy is a bold-faced lie designed to bring in dollars, and it's costing you your time, money, health, and sanity.

In a sense, this book is one long, hard truth that everyone needs to hear. If you listen, I can guarantee that you'll become physically and mentally fitter than you have ever been. You'll reach your goals. I've seen it in myself, in readers who I've turned on to Bobby's methods, and in all of the people I've met through Bobby.

If anything in this book seems like it might be harder than other methods, that's because real transformations take real effort; it's hard because it works. No, it won't always be easy. But worthwhile transformations never are.

—Michael Easter

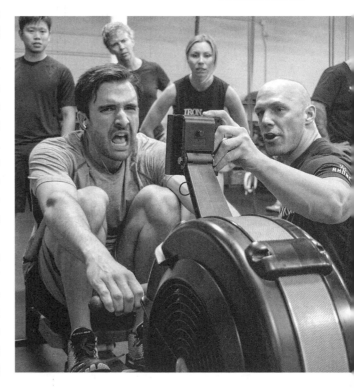

INTRODUCTION

Like many people, I came from humble beginnings. I grew up in a very small town in Northern Ontario, Canada, with two working-class parents who, more than anything else, instilled in me the value of having a strong work ethic.

I remember coming home from school as a kid with a 90 percent in math and my mother being disappointed. I was naturally gifted at math, so I never had to study. She told me that she wasn't proud of my grade because I didn't work for it. I also remember coming home with a 65 percent in geography and her telling me how proud she was because she knew I'd tried my hardest. I'd studied. The point here is that my mother never focused on the end result. She focused on the amount of work it took to get there. She noticed and rewarded work ethic. And it made me notice and reward it, too.

As I grew older, those lessons she taught me formed the basis of the person I am today.

I was never a naturally gifted athlete. In fact, I was quite the opposite. I was always the last picked for every team I tried out for, and I was bullied in elementary school and during my first few years of high school. I was uncoordinated, shy, and weak, both mentally and physically. Many of the people I've met in my lifetime have had a hard time believing that I wasn't an athlete. They look at me and make certain assumptions. They see me as supremely confident, a great speaker, and successful in all I do. The reality is that inside of me is a kid who got bullied on the bus ride to school, who was called names, and who was terrified to give public speeches.

My story of personal growth and change started when I was 14 years old. You will learn about it in the first section of this book, but without the work ethic my mother instilled in me, none of my successes would have ever happened.

Because of that work ethic, I've had many incredible life experiences. I've fought and been victorious in the Ultimate Fighting Championship, I was a highly decorated police officer in the city of Toronto, I'm directly responsible for the success of one of the very best gyms on the entire planet, Gym Jones, and I even have a shoe named after me. I remember dreaming about that when, as a child, I got my first pair of Jordans, and thinking how amazing it would be to have a shoe with my name on it. It feels even better than I imagined. Dreams can come true, but you have to work hard.

During my years as an athlete and a professional, I have worked for every accolade I have received, but don't think I didn't look for shortcuts. When you are dedicated, when you are driven and passionate, you'll look for any way to be more successful. I have bought numerous exercise books, spent more money at the nutrition store than anyone should, ordered products advertised on television, and tried every so-called magic exercise that was ever invented. I worked my ass off to find the "secret," and I am writing this book to tell you that the thing I learned is that there is no secret. There is no magic pill. You can't make three easy payments of $9.99 and hope to wake up fit. There's no easy way to get what you really want. You have to work.

Millions of people a year go through a cycle of trying to get fit, making very little progress, and regressing back to where they started. Why? They focus on the wrong things.

Some people believe that fitness is merely a physical thing. That if you simply go to the gym and eat a little better, you will achieve your goals. I believe the opposite. I believe that real, genuine fitness starts in your mind. It is one of the reasons that there is such an emphasis on psychology in this book.

If you can make your mind strong, if you can learn to hack your psychology, then getting your body fit will be easy. The most important muscle you can train sits right between your ears.

In this book, you are going to learn about psychology. Specifically, you'll learn how to:

1. **Improve your self-image.**

2. **Rid your life of excuses.**

3. **Rise above negative voices.**

4. **Work harder.**

Then you are going to learn how to train in a way that will make you successful not only in the gym but also in every other aspect of your life. You will learn how to harness the power of hard work, turn yourself into a functional athlete, and reinvent yourself, just like I did.

You're going to learn about nutrition and recovery. You will learn strategies to help you eat and

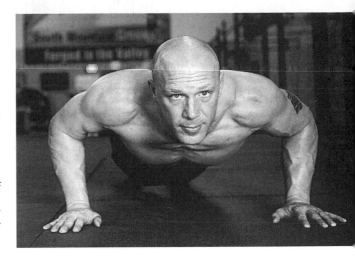

sleep better and to more effectively deal with your life stress. I'm going to help you become not only fitter but also healthier.

Throughout this book, I am going to use true stories to teach you all of these lessons. Woven into each chapter is a story of a person who has inspired me. I'll tell you about the friend or person I have been fortunate enough to work with and who has successfully used the information I am providing you with. I hope that their stories inspire you like they inspired me. I'll also share some of my personal stories and "Bobby's Laws," which I live by every day. I hope the lessons you learn here will help you to achieve the success you deserve so you can craft your own story and laws and, in turn, inspire others.

Finally, included in this book is a full training program to follow and a bank of my favorite workouts. In fact, in Section V: The Maximus Manual (see page 149), I provide you with more than 100 of the most-effective workouts in the world. They are simple but certainly not easy.

Remember that there is no easy path to your success, no shortcut, and no magic pill. But with old-fashioned hard work, and some passion for what you do, you will be successful.

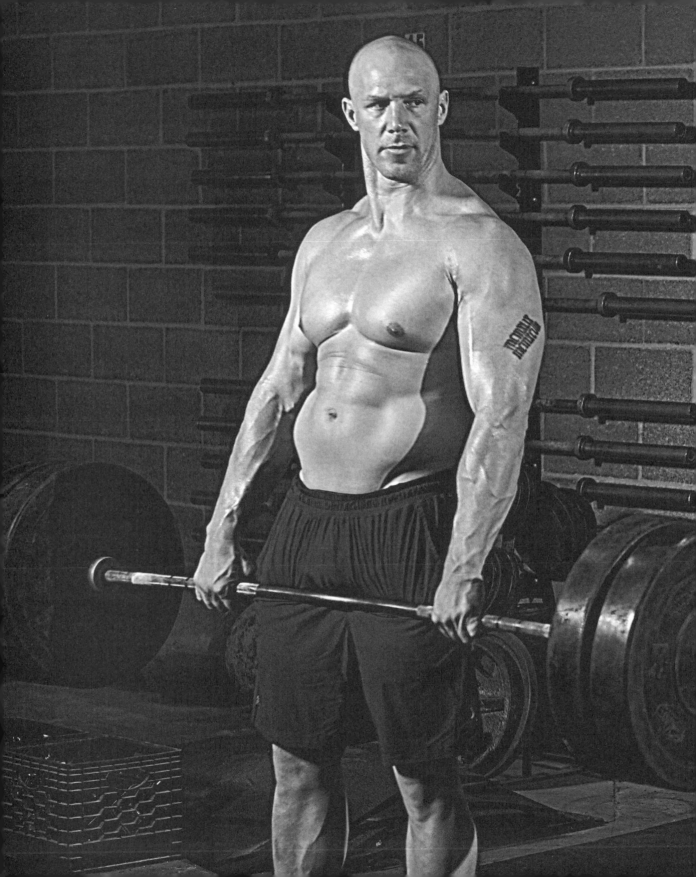

PSYCHOLOGY

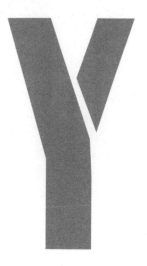

You probably think that the hardest part about exercise is the physical work: the lifting, running, and sweating. You couldn't be more wrong.

I've spent more than 20 years either as a professional athlete or as a trainer of professional athletes and special forces soldiers, and I've come to believe otherwise. Looking back on my own sports career and seeing exactly what makes the people I train successful, I've come to one conclusion: Fitness starts in your mind.

The quickest, most-effective—and, unfortunately, brutal—method I have to demonstrate that the mind is primary in fitness takes just 60 seconds. I use it on anyone who needs to quickly learn how powerful the mind can be, and I always close each of the fitness seminars I teach with the test.

Before I give the test at seminars, I ask the group—usually anywhere from 20 to 40 people—two simple questions: "Do you believe in yourself?" and "Are you willing to work hard?"

Invariably, when I ask that question, every single person says, "Yes, of course." The 1-minute fan bike challenge is the litmus test. I wheel a fan bike out into the middle of the gym floor. Then, I scribble each person's name on a big whiteboard in the gym, and jot a number next to their names.

I explain to the group: *That's how many calories each of you has to burn in 1 minute. If you don't, you try again until you do.*

Once people see the number by their names, they look terrified, like they're lining up to face a firing squad.

In general, 1 minute of jogging burns about 10 calories, a minute of weight lifting burns about 8, and a minute of yoga burns about 5. Raw, unfiltered effort on a fan bike can burn far more.

I often ask extremely fit people to burn more than 80 calories, which are calculated by the bike's computer. I even ask people of average fitness to burn 50 or more. I once asked a 65-year-old man to burn 30 calories. My personal record is 89 calories. It still hurts to think about it.

If you truly work hard and go all out in the test, you'll hit your calorie goal, or even burn a calorie or two above your goal. If you don't try hard enough, you'll fail—and there's no other excuse beyond that.

Done right, this test forces you to work harder than you ever have in your life. I've seen people vomit afterward. I've seen them hobble around dazed, jabbing at their legs for 15 minutes. I saw one guy cry, and another go outside and sit in silence for an hour afterward. (If you want to try this for yourself but you don't have a fan bike, see "What If You Don't Have a Fan Bike?" on page 4.)

You may think this test sounds cruel, but the discomfort is worth it—once the burning in your lungs and acid in your legs go away, you understand the power of hard work and feel just how valuable 1 single minute of your best effort can be. You see the number of calories you just burned in a minute, and you begin to fathom what you're capable of. Then, I hope, you start to wonder *what else can I do if I just work harder and believe in myself?*

Psychological barriers block people from reaching their goals. If you're like the vast majority of people, you probably go to the gym for one of three reasons: to become more fit to do the things you love, to become healthier, or to look better naked. For you to get in shape, you may think the answer is easy: Show up to the gym, do some exercise, and go home.

Unfortunately, it doesn't work like that. To get fit and achieve your goals, you have to do much more than just show up and slog through the motions.

We all know a person who says they work out three or four times a week but hasn't changed in 3 years. Investigate what that person actually does in a workout, and you'll usually find there is a severe lack of hard work—he texts and looks at Instagram, he only does weight exercises that feel comfortable, and if he's running, it's at a slow speed. He's probably done the same few workouts for years. If that reminds you of yourself, that's okay, because we're going to change that.

The people who become fit and stay fit are different. They don't have secret exercises or eat some "superfood," and they don't take a magic fitness pill. Above all else, they have a solid work ethic.

The most successful people show up, yes. But when they're there, they work harder than most everyone else. They believe, and they don't quit, make excuses, or take shortcuts. After their workouts, they pay attention to their fitness outside of the gym by doing other things that help them improve, like eating right and sleeping enough.

All of those habits are built by that muscle in your skull. That's precisely why training should improve your mind first. If you build a strong mind that powers hard work and dedication, then all this

HOW DO I KNOW HOW MANY CALORIES YOU CAN BURN IN A MINUTE?

When I administer the 1-minute fan-bike challenge, I give each person an individual calorie goal. So, for example, I might assign you a goal of 60 calories, while I may give your friend only 50.

How do I calculate that figure for each person? When I work with you, I notice what you do in the gym and how you do it. I pay attention to how you move weight, and how you breathe under distress. I've taken hundreds of 1-minute tests myself. My calculations are more an art than a science, but I'm rarely wrong. In fact, I'm within a calorie of the person's finishing number about 9 out of 10 times. I always set the bar exactly where it should be, and it's always higher than you think it should be.

To find your own true potential, take the test once every 2 weeks. Each time, throw yourself completely on the fire, and give it your all. Try to improve your score each time. Eventually, you'll figure out what you are capable of.

WHAT IF YOU DON'T HAVE A FAN BIKE?

The all-out minute test puts you through a mental and physical crucible that's unlike anything you've ever done. If you truly go all out, you'll come out on the other side a changed person.

I use a fan bike and give people an individual calorie target. But if you don't have a fan bike, you can see the exact same benefit from these two variations of the test. A good way to gauge if you're going hard enough is that you should want to quit about 20 seconds in, then you just have to hang on and keep going your hardest. Try it, feel some discomfort, and overcome your mental demons.

1-MINUTE SPRINT

Go to a track and set a timer for 60 seconds. When the timer starts, take off and run as fast as you possibly can until the time expires. You should aim to complete one 400-meter lap in that minute. That's well within reach for any adult male (for women, I ask for about 350 meters). If you can't do it, you have some mental work to do, even if you think it's a physical problem. To keep improving, simply go farther every time you take this test.

1-MINUTE ROW

Program a rower's timer for 1 minute, and set the screen so that it displays meters rowed. Row as hard as you can until the minute is up. Try to get as many meters as possible. Aim for a minimum of 350 meters.

"fitness stuff" is easy. Your workouts are reduced to picking shit up and putting it down, and placing one foot in front of the other.

If I only have a weekend with you—like I do with people in my fitness seminars—the fan-bike test is the best way I can demonstrate this fact.

But you and I have an entire book together. In this section, I'm going to break down four things that are paramount to getting your mind right:

▶ Improving your self-image

▶ Ridding yourself of excuses

▶ Silencing negative voices

▶ Learning why the hard road is better

The result: You'll learn why your mind is the primary driver of just how fit you can get, and you'll learn to hack your psychology to improve your body and performance across the board. Over the course of my fitness career, I've used these four rules to incite radical mental and physical changes in everyone from pro athletes to average Joes. *Real* fitness starts here.

Bobby's Law:
Decide.
Commit.
Succeed.

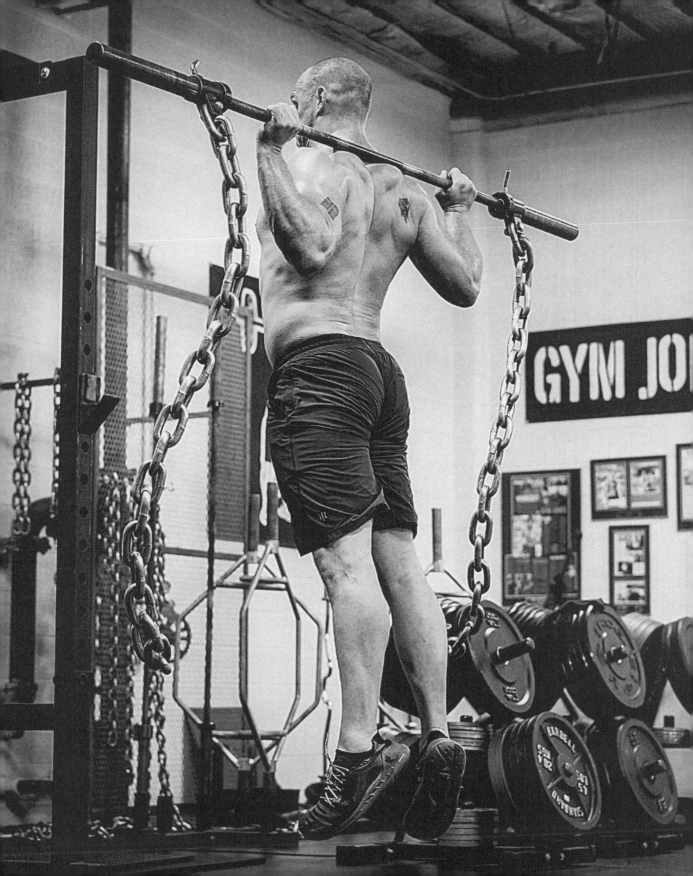

1

IMPROVE YOUR SELF-IMAGE

I'll never forget my first big fight in the Ultimate Fighting Championship (UFC). About 12,000 people crowded the sold-out Mandalay Bay Events Center in Las Vegas.

I lost that fight before the first-round bell even rang.

The reason wasn't that my nutrition was off or that I hadn't trained hard enough. In fact, I firmly believe that I'd eaten better and trained harder than not only my competition, but also any other fighter in the UFC. The reason I lost was sitting right between my ears.

I grew up in a 2,500-person northern Canadian town that's located somewhere just south of where Santa Claus lives. Even though the competition up there was slim, I was a terrible athlete. I was always the last kid picked for games in gym, and I never made the good sports teams. Bullies picked on me on the bus ride home from school every single day: They gave me wedgies, drew on my face with markers, and occasionally beat me up.

To learn to defend myself, I signed up for wrestling, which was a walk-on sport, meaning it had no try-outs. As in all athletic things, I was awful at wrestling. I lost every match my first year. The next year, I lost all but one.

Despite my losing record, I never gave up. Over those 2 years, I showed up early to every practice and decided that, even though I may not wrestle that well, I could work harder in the gym and in practice than everyone else on the team. I still wasn't winning matches, but the harder I worked, the better I became. So, the losses weren't as bad anymore.

Then, the hard work started to pay off. I began to win a lot more matches than I lost, and I became the best wrestler at my high school. After graduating high school, I went on to college and wrestled, and I was the best on that team, too.

I never lost my work ethic, kept working hard, and even branched out to other fighting sports. By the time I was 24 years old, I was a nationally ranked wrestler, an internationally ranked kick-boxer, and one of the best young mixed martial artists in Canada.

I had become a great fighter, but I still had one big, lingering disadvantage. I'd spent an incredible amount of time and effort in the gym and on the mat transforming my body and fighting skills, but I never did anything to transform my mind. I still viewed myself as the kid being drawn on and beat up. I didn't believe in myself.

Skill alone had helped me beat lesser fighters in smaller matches. But put me in a big crowd against someone as skilled as, or maybe even better than, me, and things changed. Even though my achievements and my win/loss record told me I was a winner, the 17 years of mental baggage I carried with me convinced me that I was still a loser.

I remember sitting in that Mandalay Bay dressing room thinking: *This stadium has almost five times more people than my hometown. What will people think if I lose? What will they say? I'm going to get made fun of. This guy has a better record than me; I'm going to lose. There is no way I can win. This guy fights full-time, and I have a regular job in addition to fighting. I'm going to lose. I just don't belong here.*

When I finally stepped into that ring and the bell rang, I'd already lost. My opponent submitting me in the first round was just a foregone conclusion.

I shared that story to make a simple point: You live up to who you believe you are.

If you say something is going to be hard, it will be hard. If you say you can't do something, you won't be able to do it. If you say you're bad at something, you'll do poorly. If you set your sights low, your performance will be substandard. It's as simple as that.

When you begin to truly believe in what you can do, you'll be shocked at how fast you'll improve—and how long those improvements will last.

Take me, for example. After I got my ass kicked at Mandalay Bay, I had an epiphany and realized that my negative thinking was the root of my problems. In the gym, my mindset was that of a winner. I was convinced that I could outwork any person alive, and so I did. But in the ring, it was the opposite, and I realized that I needed to fix my mind to ever be able to win a big fight. So, I began to train my brain even harder than I did my body.

Before my next UFC match—where I was a heavy underdog—I sat in that locker room preparing to fight, and it was like I had a totally new brain: My thoughts had shifted 180 degrees.

I had one of the best fights of my career. I even won submission of the night.

You'll learn the three strategies that I used leading up to that fight—strategies I use with every person I work with. These approaches will improve your mindset, helping you achieve your biggest goals in less time.

Changing thought patterns that you may have had your entire life surely won't be easy, but it's one of the greatest things you can do—not only for your fitness, but even for your general disposition. Through this process, always remember that the physical work in the gym is easy—it's just exercise. The people who are unyieldingly fit are those that have won the mental game.

Before we get down to exactly how you'll develop a winning mind-set, try a quick exercise: Identify two of the most common self-limiting beliefs that may be tying you down, just as I was. Do you see any of these in yourself?

SELF-LIMITING PATTERNS

1. You Set the Bar Too Low

The most common self-limiting pattern I see in people is having too-low expectations of them-

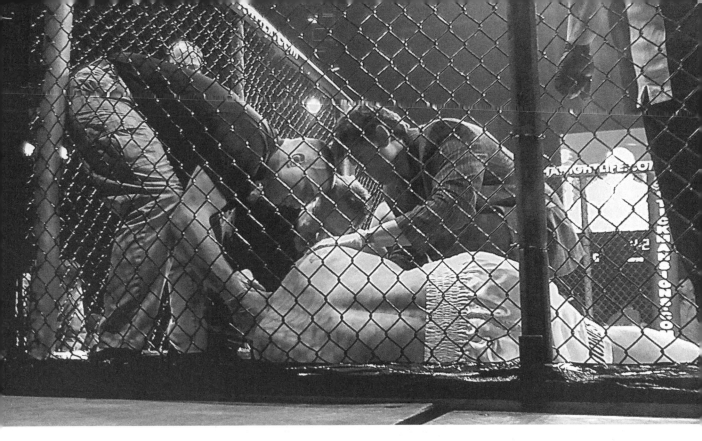

selves. Perhaps your goals are too easy. Perhaps you believe you can achieve something, but not truly big or difficult things, or anything more than average. Anytime you have a low expectation of yourself, you set a ceiling on what you're capable of—the lower your expectation, the lower your ceiling.

A good example of this is how many people approach marathons. I've met a lot of people whose ultimate goal is to finish a marathon. For them, simply crossing the finish line, they think, is the absolute best they are capable of. I like to examine that goal with a story about my favorite athlete of all time.

It was 1977, and Terry Fox's knee hurt. After ignoring the pain, he finally saw a doctor who told him that he had osteosarcoma, a rare form of cancer that often originates at the knee. Terry immediately had to have his leg amputated and, afterward, underwent 16 months of chemotherapy.

When Terry was finished with treatment, he decided he wanted to do something big to raise money for cancer research. What was "big" for Terry? Running across Canada, from east to west. To do that, he ran the equivalent of a marathon every single day for about 6 months.

Yes, Terry Fox had one leg, cancer, and he ran 26.2 miles every single day for 6 months straight.

And here you are . . . healthy, with working legs, and you're having trouble figuring out how you're going to finish just one marathon. Why not aim to do two? Why not aim to do three, or one in every state? Rather than just finish, why not give yourself a time goal?

When you do set a time goal, don't further limit yourself. I've heard countless people say their goal is to break 4 hours. Instead, why don't you try to qualify for the Boston Marathon? You've probably heard that Boston is the most difficult marathon to qualify

HOW FITNESS STANDARDS CAN SOMETIMES BRING YOU DOWN

Sometimes, what is considered to be a "good" fitness standard can actually just hold you back by setting a sort of ceiling on your potential. For example, a lot of trainers say that deadlifting double body weight is a good strength standard, or that qualifying for Boston is a good long-distance running standard. I agree, but at the same time, once people reach those standards, they often become comfortable and don't rise above them, and that holds them back from more improvement. A prime example: Ask the guy who has a deadlift world record if deadlifting double body weight is good, or the guy who won Boston if running a 3-hour marathon is good. They'd both say absolutely not. What I'm getting at is that, once you reach what you consider a good standard, don't just stay there and rest on your laurels. Either raise what you define as "good" and keep working, or find a new good standard to hit.

for. It's true: Boston has the fastest qualifying time.

But every single year, more than 25,000 people qualify. If 25,000 regular people qualify, why can't you? What's stopping you?

Believe in yourself. Set your standards high. You are capable. I know you can be one of those qualifiers for Boston, or any other event that you want to excel in, because I see it every day in the people I work with.

2. You Think That You're a Special Case

I had an interesting conversation with a middle-aged woman who was about 30 pounds overweight. When I mentioned that I work in the fitness industry, she told me that she'd briefly tried a couple trainers and eating plans in order to lose weight, but that she hadn't been successful.

She went on to explain, "Genetically, I just have a slower metabolism and am just a heavier person. I'll always be heavy because my body wants me to be at this weight."

I didn't say anything because she didn't hire me to coach her, but if she had hired me, I would have had some news for her. You are not special, you are not a unique snowflake, and your excuses are bullshit. I don't care who you are: If you work out regularly and eat appropriately, you are capable of losing weight.

Yes, you may have to do a little work to find what diet works for you or hire an expert nutritionist, and you'll have to work hard in the gym. But if you do those two things, you will lose weight. Do you honestly think you defy biology and are the only one in the world who is incapable of losing weight?

I don't mean to sound harsh, but I don't bullshit the people I work with. Indulging an incorrect "I'm-special" thought pattern does a disservice to everyone.

This "I'm-special" phenomenon occurs in many other areas as well. Have you ever heard phrases like "I just can't get strong," "I'm too tall to do pull-ups," or "I'm naturally not a good runner."

These are all self-limiting beliefs. If you say you aren't or can't, then you are not and cannot.

Usually, these excuses are formed from your experience. Perhaps you failed at things in the past, and those failures have stayed at the back of your mind, telling you that you're "bad" and negatively affecting your self-image. No one likes to look bad, but you can't look good and improve at the same time. No one looks good when they're learning. In fact, it takes courage to learn. You have to accept that it's part of the process.

Or, perhaps you're comparing yourself to someone. Maybe your brother, for example, was a state champion runner, and you've spent your entire life comparing your running times to his. Yeah, you may never top the 4:00-mile time that he set in high school. But you can still improve your running, be the best version of yourself, and excel in local races.

Don't get me wrong; there are some physical limitations that are more difficult to overcome, and there are certain physical attributes that make certain tasks relatively easier. For example, taller guys are usually better on the rowing machine, and people with short arms tend to be better at bench press. Lighter people are often better at body-weight movements.

But just because you have a certain build or genetics doesn't mean that you should accept that you're bad at something. I truly believe that with enough work you can be good at anything you put your mind to. No, you may not be the best in the world, but you can break into the top 90 percentile of any skill by believing in yourself and working hard. I see it in the people I work with every single day.

HOW TO FREE YOURSELF OF SELF-IMPOSED LIMITATIONS

The simple reality is that you're just going to be spinning your wheels, sabotaging yourself, and going nowhere unless you can learn to fix your head and break free of your self-imposed limitations. The big question is: *How do I do that?* It certainly isn't easy. It will take some time and attention. But the payoffs are beyond anything that an individual exercise, diet, or supplement can deliver.

I've found that the following three strategies are successful for everyone that I work with. In fact, they're the same exact strategies that I used after that Mandalay Bay fight, and the same ones I've used to help thousands of people reach incredible fitness. They'll shift your thinking to that of a winner and allow you to be more successful than you ever imagined.

1. Think "Green-Light Thoughts"

Self-doubt kills your performance, and self-doubt begins in your mind, with your mental dialogue—so change that dialogue, and your performance will change.

After I lost my fight at Mandalay Bay, something clicked, and I realized that my negative thoughts and self-talk are what may have held me back from winning. So, I sought out a professional who could help me improve.

The very first thing my sports psychologist, Brian Cain, had me do was to sort my thoughts into

THE 8 BEST PLACES TO PUT GREEN DOTS

A good place to put positive-thought-boosting green dots is anywhere you'll see them most often. The more you see the green dots, the more positive self-talk you will engage in. The more positive self-talk you engage in, the quicker you will be able to reprogram your brain. Here are the spots to place them:

1. Cell phone
2. Refrigerator
3. Water bottle
4. Gym bag
5. Steering wheel
6. Computer
7. Barbell
8. Favorite exercise machine

"red-light thoughts" and "green-light thoughts."

Red-light thoughts are inherently negative thoughts. They tell you all the reasons why you can't do something. For example, *I have poor genetics, I don't belong here, I am not a strong person,* and *I know a lot of people who have failed.* These were the exact same types of thoughts I had in the dressing room before my losing fight.

Green-light thoughts, on the other hand, are positive thoughts that breed success. They sound like this: *There are others who are successful, I know I can be, too; I belong here, I am capable of this;* and *Nobody works harder than I do.*

The more red-light thoughts you think, the more likely you are to develop a negative self-image—and the more likely you are to fail. The more green-light thoughts you think, the more likely you are to succeed.

Cain has worked with thousands of athletes and proved, time and time again, that green-light thoughts push your performance forward and induce success.

Everyone has a balance of the two. No one is immune to self-doubt, but you need to learn to shift your thinking to tip the balance in favor of green-light thoughts.

To do that, I placed little green stickers over the places I frequented the most: on my car's steering wheel, on the bathroom mirror, inside the fridge, and on the weight rack. Every time I saw one of those green dots, I told myself one reason that I was going to succeed and reach my goal. This constant repetition of positive thoughts shifted my thinking and made me think about myself positively. After a few weeks of simply thinking green-light thoughts every single time I saw a green dot, I began to see myself as a person who wins big UFC fights.

When I sat in the dressing room for my next fight, guess what I was thinking? Green-light

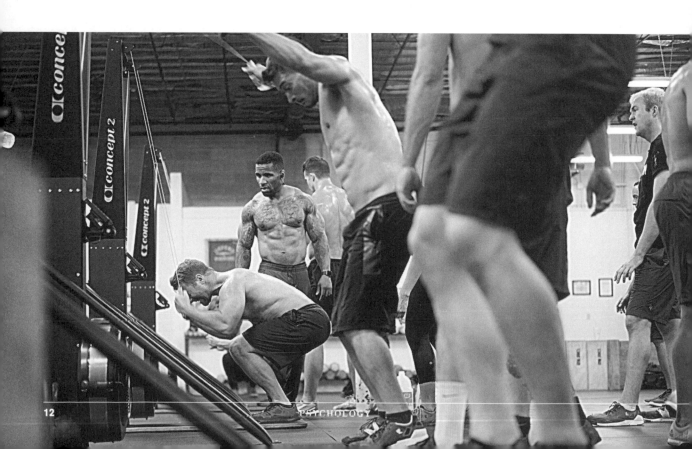

PSYCHOLOGY

THREE THINGS I STILL STRUGGLE WITH

1. SPEAKING IN PUBLIO

When I was in school, speaking in public terrified me. I'd stutter and struggle to remember words, and it made me think that I looked stupid and I wondered what others thought of me. I've improved over the years, but I still get nervous to lead a seminar, even though I've taught hundreds of them. Sometimes, I get so nervous that I want to throw up before, especially if it's one with a lot of people. When this happens, I take 5 minutes and do some positive self-talk, reminding myself that I'm great at leading seminars and that it will go well. It always helps quell my butterflies. Do the same. Take 5 minutes to sit and visualize your speech going well, and use positive self-talk.

2. TESTING A LIFT

The deadlift is my strongest lift, but I often doubt myself before testing a 1-rep max. I don't think I'm strong enough, or I worry that I'll hurt my back. To fix this, I use music. In training, I pick a song that motivates me. Each time I go hard in training, I listen to that song. When it's time to deadlift, I play that song, and it helps me remember all of the hard work and the successes I've had before, forget about my doubts, and just lift hard and heavy. Do the same or use some other cue that works for you.

3. HAVING BUSINESS MEETINGS

Training people is only a fraction of my job. A major part of my job is running a successful brand. I regularly engage in meetings with professional athletes, CEOs, agents, and representatives of big businesses. I'm not always confident; we're a small gym, and we often have to work with multimillion-dollar entities. But, I've found that by acting confident, I am able to make better choices, I am able to do better in the business meeting, and I am able to be better at my job. Before a meeting, I always repeat to myself: *Let your actions dictate your feelings. Don't let your feelings dictate your actions.* That reminds me that confidence breeds success.

thoughts: *I'm going to win, I've trained so hard for this that there's no way I can't win, I'm way more fit than this guy,* and *I'm going to win this easily.* I was right.

I suggest that you do the same. Whether your goal is to lose 20 pounds, run a fast 5K, or double your strength, place green dots in the places that you see most often (you can buy the dots at an office supply store).

You can even use this trick in training. In the past, for example, I've placed a green dot on a rower for people who were letting negative self-talk sabotage their efforts during a 2,000-meter rowing test.

Instead of thinking *I'm too tired* or *I need to slow down,* it helped people to tell themselves that *I've got this, I'm going to crush this, This is easy,* and *I feel great.* This positive self-talk reinforces your confi-

dence and improves your output, essentially overriding your brain's performance-crushing negativity.

2. Write Down 5 Reasons Why You'll Succeed

When you write something down, it becomes real.

As I was trying to reprogram my self-image and deal with my limitations in the ring, I woke up every morning and began my day by writing down five reasons why I was going to succeed.

It's a simple yet extremely powerful exercise. At some point each day, write down five reasons why you're going to accomplish your goal. Don't overcomplicate it—your reasons can be the same every day. Or you could come up with different explanations. It really doesn't matter. What does

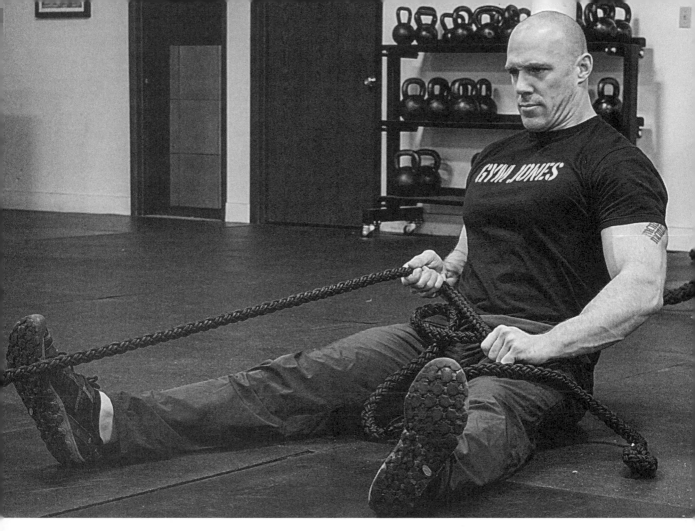

matter is that this practice forces you to cognitively recognize and process all the good you're doing every single day.

As an example, let's say you're trying to qualify for the Boston Marathon. A day's entry might look like this:

1. I haven't missed a single run since I started my training.
2. Injuries are the biggest reason runners become sidetracked, and I haven't had a single ache or pain.
3. Yesterday, I ran 10 seconds faster than the qualifying mile pace for 18 miles straight. Twenty-six miles will be easy.
4. Running the qualifying pace feels easy to me. I can do it forever.
5. I am training harder than I ever have in my life. I will be successful.

3. Visualize Success

Every day after my losing fight, I watched a DVD containing highlights of my best moments as a fighter and athlete. It helped me see what winning and success look like and helped me change my negative self-image. This was a form of visualization.

Visualization was used heavily by Soviet sports

scientists in the 1970s, and it's something a large number of professional athletes and businessmen at the top of their games use today. Visualization is simple: You take time each day to psychologically rehearse what you want to accomplish, like you're the main character in a movie that is playing in your mind.

So, let's say your goal is to run a mile in under 6 minutes. You'd mentally picture and rehearse exactly what you need to do to accomplish that feat. You'd think of yourself running on the track where you intend to test yourself, imagining yourself feeling great as you held pace, breathed easy, and ran fast. The more details you incorporate, the more effective visualization is.

Yes, this may sound a little far out, but pro athletes ranging from Jack Nicklaus to Muhammad Ali to Kobe Bryant have used this technique with great success.

Science confirms that visualization has tangible performance-enhancing benefits. Consider this study[1] by researchers at the Cleveland Clinic: People who visualized doing a strength-training exercise for 15 minutes a day, 5 days a week, for 12 weeks (but didn't actually lift) increased their strength by anywhere from 13.5 to 35 percent.

Scientists believe visualization works by altering processes in your brain, like your motor control, attention, perception, planning, and memory, while also enhancing your motivation and confidence. So, when it comes time to perform, in your mind, you've already won—your brain is "trained" for the actual performance and success.

Bobby's Law:
The bar is never set high enough. Always look to raise it.

For visualization to work, you need to take it seriously and be fully committed. Here's how the process should go: Every day, sit somewhere quiet and close your eyes. Free yourself of all other extraneous thoughts. Take deep breaths and simply think about exactly what you'll need to do to reach your goal—visualize your surroundings and engage all of your senses. Do it for 5 to 15 minutes, 5 days a week.

If you think this sounds weird, ask yourself a question: Could it hurt? Little things like this are what make the difference between winners and losers. It only takes a few moments a day, and it could be the thing that leads you to success.

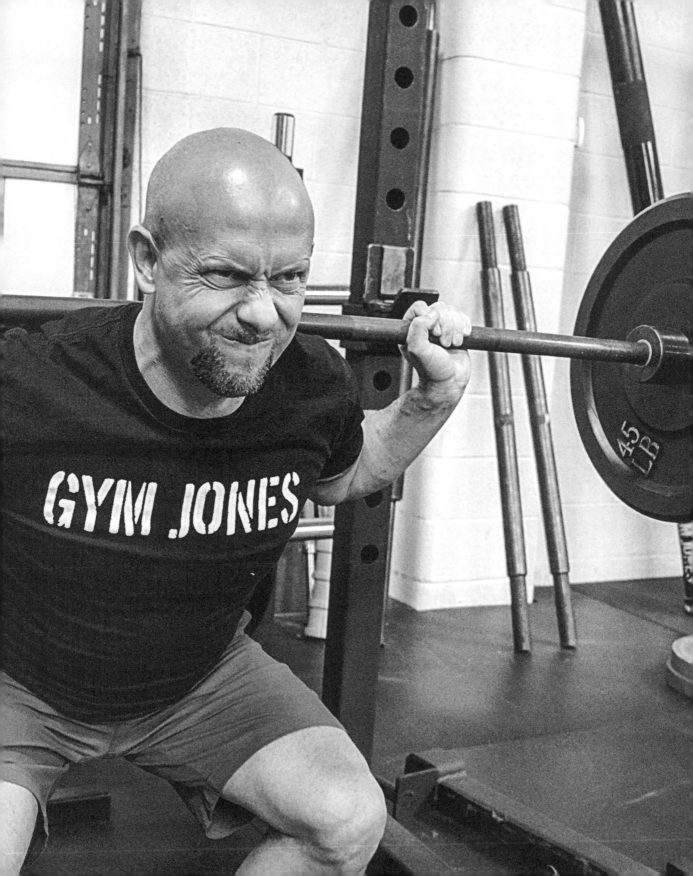

2

DON'T MAKE EXCUSES

Preston Wood is 44 years old and was never a natural athlete. He's not a big guy, standing just 5'6" and weighing 158 pounds. He works often, usually logging anywhere from 60 to 70 hours a week, and his job demands a lot of travel. He also has a wife and family that he puts above all else and lives in a town that is about an hour-and-a-half round-trip from our gym.

I've heard people use all of those reasons—work, family, small stature, age, time—as an excuse to not become fit. But Preston is one of the fittest guys who comes to Gym Jones—despite his so-called limitations, he's reached a truly incredible level of fitness, for anyone, of any age or size.

I've never been easy on Preston. I give him the most difficult of standards to achieve. I don't give him a break because of his height, weight, work schedule, or age. Despite that, he hits all of the fitness standards that I ask him to achieve and always goes above and beyond.

The reason Preston is so fit is simple: When it's time to work, Preston always works his hardest, and he never makes excuses. Yes, Preston *could* make a lot of excuses for why he can't train or can't perform in the gym. But he doesn't—Preston rarely misses a gym session. And if he does, he always makes it up by doing a workout at home.

Preston is one of the greatest excuse-killers for the other people I train—he's a litmus test for bullshit. When anyone else tells me that they don't have time to achieve their goals because of their work, family, commute, or because they just aren't suited for something, I can say, "Well, Preston works more than you. He also has a family. He lives farther away from the gym than you. He's also older and smaller than you. But Preston does it. Why can't you?"

Among the people I work with, the word "Preston" is the ultimate excuse-killer.

Sure, every day isn't easy for Preston. There are days he fails, just like the rest of us. He's human. But what makes him unique is that when he does fail, he always tries harder the next time. He never indulges me or himself with excuses. He analyzes his failure and fixes what went wrong. I once asked him why he never makes excuses. His answer: "Excuses indicate mental weakness. When you use an excuse, you're telling yourself and others that you aren't willing to take any personal responsibility to either accept or change an outcome."

Be like Preston. Don't make excuses—taking ownership of your failures is one of the most important things you can do if you're ever going to become fit and reach your goals. When people don't reach a goal—or are so afraid of failure that they don't even try—they often make excuses. "I didn't have enough time," "I didn't have the right exercise program," or "My nutrition was off." The list goes on and on. As a trainer, I've heard some pretty absurd ones.

Excuses are a coping mechanism. They are your mind's way of trying to rationalize why you fail so you feel better. Don't let excuses fly. When you fail, learn from it, fix the problem, and try again—this time harder. Reaching a goal is as simple as applying effort consistently and deliberately, while getting rid of all the additional bullshit.

I use a simple drill with people who make too many excuses. Every time you find yourself making an excuse for why you didn't perform well or failed, I want you to stop yourself and say, "I won't make excuses, I will try harder." This helps you recognize a negative thought pattern, and it motivates you to give more effort. Be accountable and honest with yourself. Use this technique, and use it often.

It's also worthwhile to tackle the two most common excuses that I hear: "I don't have enough time" and "I don't have fitness equipment." When people say these to me, we have a conversation wherein I analyze their claims. This conversation is so powerful that you and I need to have it too.

THESE EXCUSES DON'T FLY

1. I don't have enough time.

The single most common excuse I hear from people is "I don't have enough time to work out." When people feed me that line, we fill out one of my infamous time audits.

In this exercise, the person claiming this and I stand in front of a big whiteboard. I write "168" in big numbers. I tell the person that 168 happens to be the number of hours there are in a week.

Then, I ask the person how many hours he works and sleeps each week. For the purpose of this exercise, let's say he works 70 hours a week—that's 14 hours each day, Monday through Friday. Then, I usually assign the person 8 hours of sleep each night, or 56 weekly hours. I don't ask about sleep, I tell—people rarely get 8 hours of sleep every night, but that's how much they *should* be sleeping (which is something we'll address later).

Add 70 and 56, and the person has used only 126 hours out of a possible 168. Do the math, and we're left with 42 extra *waking* hours each week that this guy tells me he "doesn't" have. That's the equivalent of nearly 2 days that he claims just aren't there. I ask the person what the hell he does with the rest of his time. It's a fair question.

The person inevitably starts to shout things like "I have to commute to work," "I have to grocery shop," and "I have to spend time with my family!"

So without even asking him, I give the guy 10 hours of commuting (2 hours, 5 days a week), 3 hours of weekly grocery shopping, and 20 hours of quality time with his family.

That brings his total hours to 159 hours, meaning he still has 9 hours each week. By now, the guy gets the message.

Everyone has enough time for health and fitness. If you choose not to use it, that's your prerogative. But realize that it is not a question of *can't*—it

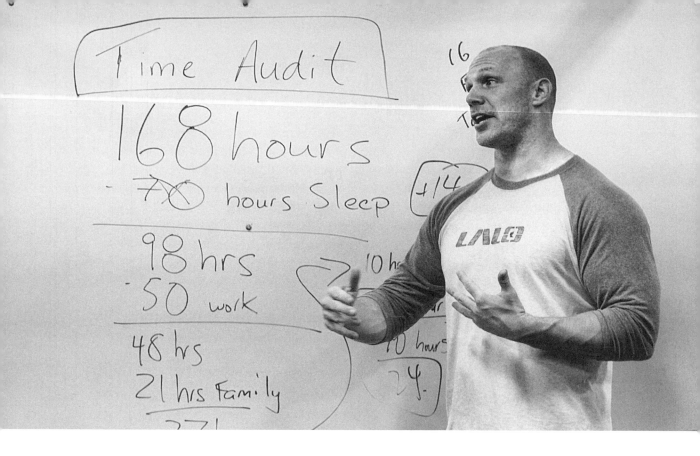

is a *choice*. I understand that there are some days when things come up, and you really may not have time to train that day. But, over the course of a week, you do have the time.

Whenever I do this exercise with a person, I always think of my friend Casey. Casey is a trader on Wall Street whose schedule is a lot like the one above: He works 14-hour days, Monday through Friday. He also has a newborn and a long commute. If anyone doesn't have enough time, it's this guy.

Despite that, Casey never misses a training session. He goes to bed at 9:00 so that he can get up at 4:30 every morning, and he is in the gym working his ass off while most people are asleep. That work

RUN YOUR OWN TIME AUDIT

Right now, I want you to try this drill. Grab a pen and paper. Write how many estimated weekly hours you work, sleep, commute, shop, and spend with your loved ones. If you want, add in a weekly amount of time you spend doing other activities that you think are important. I don't care what this is. It could be walking your dog, watching your favorite sports, or a hobby, like woodworking.

Add all those numbers up. Now, take that number and subtract it from 168. The result is how many extra hours you have each week that you could spend reaching your goal.

Hopefully, you get it now, too.

Bobby's Law:
Sometimes you are the hammer. Other times, you are the nail.

ethic has allowed him to become an absolute machine. The guy can row well below a sub-7-minute 2,000-meter row and deadlift far more than double his body weight. More importantly, Casey says the time he devotes in the gym allows him to be more productive at work, and a better father.

In truth, Casey's schedule is a rarity. The funniest thing about this exercise is that most people who say they don't have enough time to train don't work 70 hours a week, don't sleep 8 hours a night, don't commute 2 hours a day, and don't spend that much time with their family. So, in reality, they have significantly more than 9 hours each week to train. I've actually heard the "not enough time" claim from people who don't even have a job. Where does all their extra time go?

If you somehow *still* really think that you don't have the time to train, you need to question your commitment. What are you choosing over health and fitness? Facebook? Instagram? Your favorite television show? Unfortunately, I can't run another audit that helps you to realize that your commitment is what is lacking. Commitment, willpower, and motivation have to come from within. I can't force you to train or do the exercises for you. That's on you.

2. I don't have fitness equipment.

The other excuse I hear is, "I don't have fitness equipment."

I train a lot of special forces soldiers—men who put their lives on the line and make incredible sacrifices for our freedom. The job requires an incredibly high level of fitness. They need to be able to cover expansive distances while carrying heavy

WHAT IF YOU HAVE KIDS?

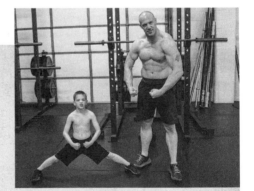

Sorry, that's not an excuse either. I've been a father for 8 years, and I don't think I've missed one workout because of my son.

How'd I do it?

▶ I'd work out in my garage. My son would come into the garage with me and play with his toys.

▶ I bought a membership to a gym that had a daycare for my son to hang out in.

▶ I'd do pushups and squats in the living room as my son watched his favorite movies for the hundredth time.

All you have to do is get a little creative. I once heard about a guy who went through four sets of wheels on a running stroller because he didn't use his kid as an excuse to cut down on his running training.

On a bigger level, when you exercise around your kid, you're demonstrating good fitness behavior. In fact, now, when my son and I watch movies together, he'll often join me for sets of pushups and squats.

THE REPETITION GRID: MY FAVORITE NO-EQUIPMENT, NO TIME WORKOUT

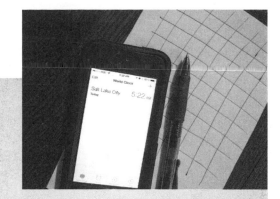

I work in a gym, and some days, even I don't have much time for a workout. So, between phone calls, training people, business development, and working with interning instructors, I find creative ways to sneak in exercise.

That's where my rep grid workouts come into play. It's a smart way to pack a ridiculous amount of valuable reps into your day without ever breaking a sweat. Do it: Before your day starts, get a piece of paper and draw a 10-by-10-square grid. Then, pick a body-weight exercise you can do anywhere. My favorite is pushups, but you could also do squats, lunges, or even pullups. Whenever you have a spare moment, perform a few reps (don't ever max out). Mark that number in one of the boxes.

Repeat throughout the day until your grid is filled, then add the numbers up. You'll be amazed how many reps you did. Even if you do just 3 reps each mini set, you'll accumulate 300 total reps. That's more than most people do in a month.

loads—a bagful of weapons, explosives, and medical and communications gear—and also need to powerfully breach enemy compounds, and come out on top in hand-to-hand combat.

Sometimes, these soldiers are deployed to areas where they have access to some gym equipment. But, more often than not, they don't have any gear to train with. No barbells and plates, no rower or fan bike or even a single dumbbell. When these soldiers are faced with this problem, do you think they throw up their hands and say "I can't work out because I don't have equipment," and then simply stop training and let their fitness levels slide?

No, they do not. Special forces soldiers have no choice but to figure out a way to stay in peak physical condition. For them, fitness can literally be a matter of life and death—train or die.

Despite their equipment limitations, they always manage to stay in extremely good shape and sometimes even improve their fitness. They do body-weight exercises or use whatever is convenient as a load. I know soldiers who have used a backpack and rocks as a weight-lifting tool.

If a special forces soldier—some of whom are the fittest guys on the planet—doesn't need fancy equipment to get fit, I can guarantee you that you don't, either. (In fact, in Section V: The Maximus Manual [see page 149], you'll find 16 no-gear workouts, many of which I give to special forces soldiers.)

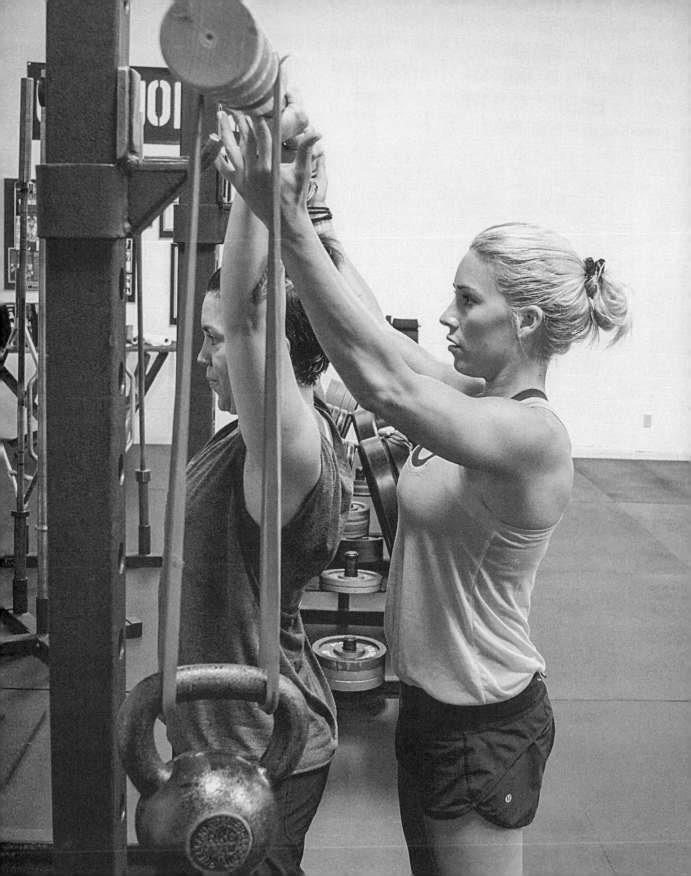

3

RISE ABOVE

A few years ago, I worked with a girl named Danielle, who came to me with a clear goal: to run a marathon in 4 hours or less.

Danielle's work ethic was incredible. She showed up early to every gym session, always went above and beyond what was expected of her, never made excuses, and was willing to put 15 quality hours a week into her training.

Building endurance is about one thing: putting in a lot of quality miles and time—there are no shortcuts. That's because to build a solid endurance base, you need to keep your heart rate elevated for an extended period of time. Keep your heart rate high enough, for long enough, and you'll progress and perform well. If not, you simply won't finish with a fast time in your race.

Danielle was well on her way to being successful. She was willing to put in the hours. She was willing to do the work. She believed in herself.

But when Danielle shared her goal with some of her coworkers, her situation changed. They told her that running a sub-4-hour marathon would be the hardest thing she'd ever do, and that she probably wouldn't reach her goal. They told her that they'd tried to run a marathon and that finishing in

4 hours or less was an impossible goal for a normal girl like her with a full-time job.

After that, Danielle heard her coworkers' voices on all her training runs, and she began to wonder if her goal was too optimistic. She worried about what they'd think and say if she failed. Her confidence began to evaporate, and she came to believe that her goal was too optimistic.

Danielle decided that maybe finishing in 4:30 was more realistic for her, in light of what her coworkers had told her. She was pretty sure she could do that—and when she announced her change of mind, her coworkers were happy to hear that she'd adopted the lesser goal.

From then on, no surprise, Danielle's running performance suffered. Runs that were once easy now felt difficult. She began to live down to the new expectations she'd set for herself.

When Danielle checked in with me to talk about her training, I was shocked. All of her times were significantly slower than just a few weeks before. When I asked her what was going on, she explained to me that 4 hours was going to be too hard. She told me about the conversations she had had with her coworkers, how all of them had failed to achieve the same goal, and how she felt that she was better off setting a lower goal.

Garbage, I told her. Based on her fitness level and how dedicated she was to training, I explained, there was actually no reason that she couldn't run significantly *faster* than a 4-hour marathon. In fact, I told Danielle, she was actually more likely to run closer to a 3-hour marathon. Then, I gave Danielle some homework: I told her to ask her coworkers about how hard they had trained for their marathons.

A couple of days later, Danielle came to me with some troubling facts. Chief among them was that most of her coworkers had only trained between 3 and 5 hours each week for their marathons. Danielle was training anywhere from 3 to 5 times more than these people, yet they wanted her to believe that she was on the same level as them.

I told Danielle that it was no surprise that her coworkers had a hard time running a marathon—they simply hadn't put in the required amount of work. Despite our conversation, it seemed the damage was already done—after another week's check-in, Danielle's times were still slower.

After thinking about how I could convince Danielle that she was capable of being a great marathoner, it dawned on me that I shouldn't be the one to convince her. After all, I've never run a marathon—what kind of advice could I really offer? So, I turned her over to a group who could convince her that she *was* capable of more: I told her to join a local running club, comprised of serious runners.

The people in Danielle's running group delivered a complete opposite message compared to her coworkers. Her new friends were positive and encouraging, and their standards were high. They told Danielle that 4-hour marathons were for people who didn't train that hard. They told her that, given her fitness level, drive, and how much time she was willing to devote to training, she was probably capable of running a 3-hour marathon.

It was amazing how quickly Danielle improved once she had positive voices that she believed in her ear. Her training-run times dropped immediately. She told me that she felt more confident, and believed that she was going to crush her goal time of 4 hours. And, when Danielle eventually did run her marathon, she ran so fast that she was able to qualify for the Boston Marathon.

There will never be a shortage of people who have failed to achieve their fitness goals. They tried to lose 20 pounds and failed. They tried to get stronger and failed. They tried to run a marathon in a certain time and failed.

Failing is okay, but it's unacceptable to put that expectation of failure on others. There are people who, when they fail, will discourage others from achieving the same goals. When people tell you how hard your goal will be, that you will fail, or that you need to find a new goal, they're doing you a true disservice. These kinds of people may not be doing it intentionally, but they are hurting your ability to succeed.

The truth is, when a person doesn't achieve their fitness goal, there is only one person they can blame: themselves.

This might sound harsh, but it's the truth. And on the bright side, there's also a great promise in that, a promise that is the core of why I love fitness so much.

Fitness is the only area of life where effort is guaranteed to produce results. In other areas of life, that isn't true, and you can simply run into bad luck: You could be the perfect husband or wife, and your partner could be unfaithful. You could run your business perfectly, and the economy could tank and your business could close. You could drive perfectly safely, and someone could run a red light and smash into you. So much of life is out of our hands.

Fitness isn't out of your hands. If you work hard enough in the gym, you will always achieve your goal. It's a very basic contract: If you do A, you'll get B. The gym is one of the only places in the world where hard work guarantees success.

Always remember that basic premise when you're working to achieve a fitness-based goal. Never let other people convince you otherwise. Just like Danielle, you'll struggle with negative voices and wonder what others think. Everyone does. I know I have.

When people, including myself, are having a hard time blocking out negative voices, I have

three methods I use to leverage the power of a positive community to reach a goal.

1. SURROUND YOURSELF WITH POSITIVE PEOPLE

You can't choose your family, but you can choose who you spend your time with. Danielle would never have qualified for the Boston Marathon had she not traded her negative-minded coworkers for a much more positive, supportive peer group.

If you surround yourself with people who

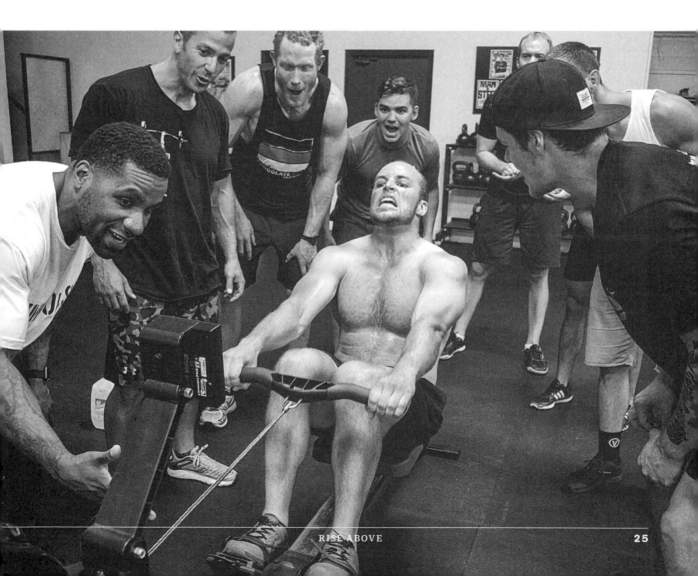

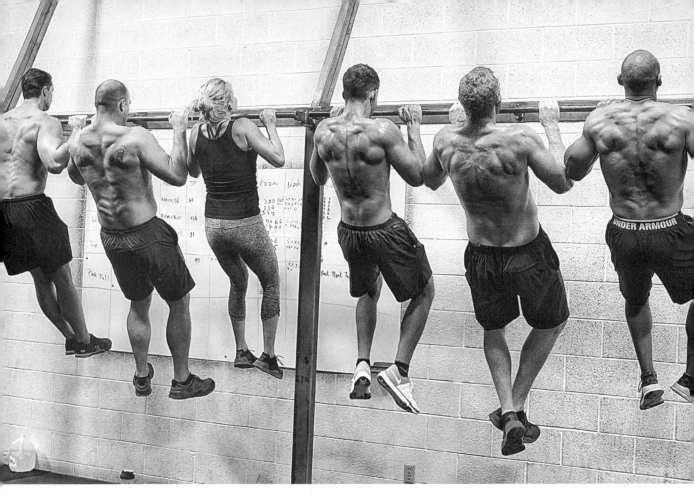

inspire you, who are better than you, who work harder and are more dedicated than you, the same will happen to you as happened to Danielle. You will improve and exceed your expectations.

Why? Being in the midst of success is an incredible motivator: It tells you exactly what is possible. In working with fit people, you'll be focused on keeping up with the group and less on your own limitations. Confidence breeds confidence, and success breeds success. The reverse is also true: Doubt breeds doubt, and failure breeds failure.

Surround yourself with the right people, and finding your way to success will be easier.

2. AVOID THESE 10 WORDS

Negative voices from other people don't just come from their mouths, they also come from your own head.

In my opinion, the 10 most dangerous words in the English language are: "What will other people think, what will other people say?"

We've all worried about how we're perceived by others. It's human nature. You probably realize that you shouldn't care what others think and say about you, because it really does not matter. But, it's far easier said than done.

Even when people don't have anything to say or don't care, we assume they do. We can sabotage ourselves in this way—how often have you not done something or underperformed only because you were too preoccupied wondering about other peoples' perception of you? The truth is that the reason most people don't care about anything you do is because they're too busy worrying about what *you're* thinking about *them*!

Personally, I used to care far too much about what others thought or said about me. The truth was that the majority of that fear was manufactured in my own head. For example, as I sat in that Mandalay Bay dressing room, I worried what other police officers back home would think if I lost the fight. But when I got back home after losing that fight, my fellow officers actually congratulated me for fighting at such a high level.

Over time, I found a solution to my problem. I found great solace in simply telling myself: *The 10 most dangerous words in the English language are: What will other people think, what will other people say?* It reminds me that clinging to the thoughts of others is only going to bring me down. By doing this, I'm able to focus more on working hard and getting better so I can reach my goals.

Develop your own mantra that you use to get out of your own head. It should remind you that what other people think ultimately isn't important. You can use mine, or you can make up your own. Whenever you find yourself thinking about another person's judgment of you, repeat it.

3. ANNOUNCE YOUR GOAL

There are few motivators stronger than accountability. Being accountable to someone you trust and respect—as opposed to fearing judgment from others—compels you to work harder. I see it every day, and I saw it, for example, in Danielle's

HOW CAN YOU FIND THE RIGHT GYM?

Certain gym atmospheres are more conducive to certain goals. Why? They're filled with like-minded individuals, all equally focused on similar goals. Everyone constantly pushes each other to improve. There's a reason, for example, that I had Danielle join a running group and not do her run days with me—I'm slow over the long haul, and the people in her run group were fast, which showed her what was possible.

Here are a few different gym atmospheres that may put you in a position to reach your goal faster.

To become strong: Power lifters have one primary goal: to become as strong as possible. Find a powerlifting federation in your geographic region, e-mail its president, and ask if he knows of any gyms close to you.

To run a marathon: Look for a running group in your area. Local specialty running stores often host a group or weekly run night.

To get generally fit: Train anywhere, but try to find a training partner. Friendly competition will push you to work harder. Can't find a training partner? Seek out a good CrossFit box. Find a list of CrossFit affiliates near you at crossfit.com.

To lose weight: Here, the gym doesn't matter so much as what you're putting in your mouth. If you have a hard time sticking to the nutrition rules you learn in this book, consider hiring a nutritionist who will keep you accountable.

relationship to her running group. They knew she was capable of more, and they let her know it. They believed in her. They held her accountable. If she ever half-assed a run, they were there to cheer her on or help her get to the bottom of why her training was off.

When we are in a group of people that hold us accountable, more often than not we rise to the occasion because we don't want to let people that we trust and respect down. That's why, whenever I have a new goal, I announce it to people that I know will support me: the people I train with and my wife. I tell them what I want to accomplish and exactly how I plan to do it. By voicing my goal to my inner circle, it makes it real.

Find a person or two that you trust, and do the same thing. You could also always make a public announcement on your Facebook.

HOW SOCIAL MEDIA CAN INSPIRE YOU TO LOSE WEIGHT

I've never met Jon Orton. We've only communicated through social media, but Jon has inspired me beyond belief.

In 2 years, Jon has gone from weighing 478 pounds to weighing 234 pounds. That's a loss of 244 pounds—the guy literally lost more than he weighs right now. He did it through changing every aspect of his life. He began to eat incredibly healthy, practice jiu jitsu, and train in power lifting and endurance. He tracked his journey on social media and was motivated by, and also inspired by, a hell of a lot of people along the way.

You may be surprised to hear it, but I've used social media to reach goals myself. Social media can be a powerful motivational tool when you are connected with a group of like-minded, supportive people. I'll often announce my goals on social media, and the friends I've made there motivate me to train hard.

In fact, a study[2] conducted by researchers at the University of Massachusetts Medical School found that you can get a lot of beneficial fitness accountability and encouragement from places on the internet, particularly forums and through social media.

Sure, sometimes there are negative people on social media, but just block them out. If you open your eyes, you'll find positive people all over. Seek them out. Learn from them.

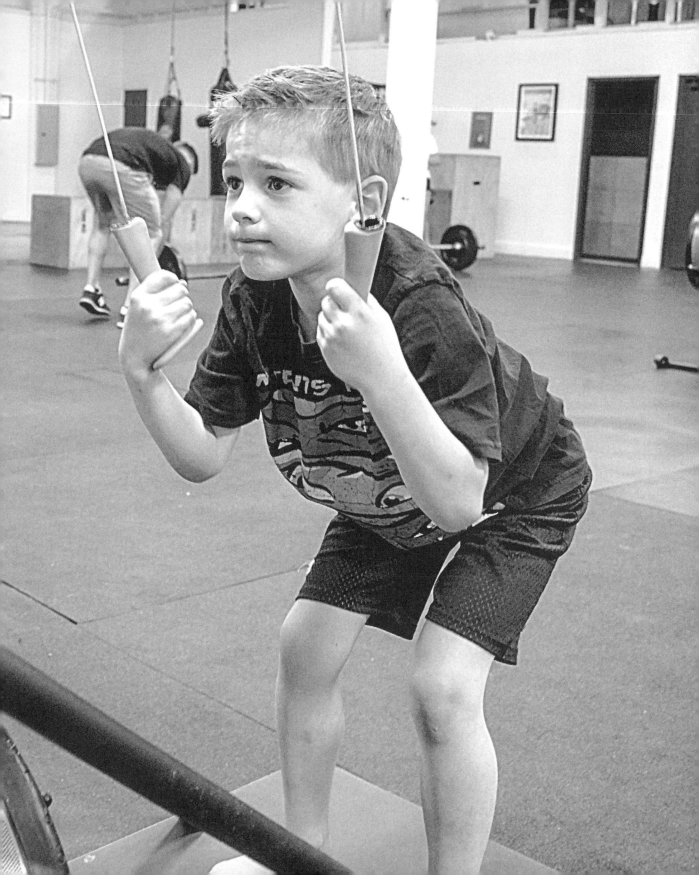

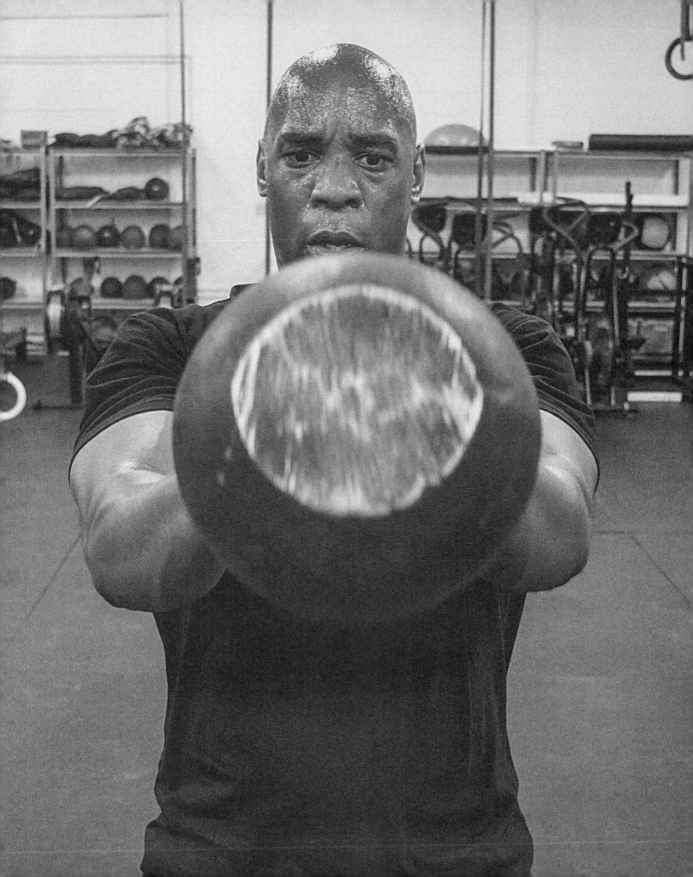

DO WHAT'S RIGHT, NOT WHAT'S EASY

As a society, we've been conditioned to think that getting fit not only doesn't take much time but is incredibly easy. You're inundated with infomercials and fitness products that promise you results:

> "Build sculpted, rock-hard abs in less than 8 minutes a day!"

> "Hate dieting? Lose weight fast and eat the foods you love with the Cookie Diet!"

> "Never work out again. Build a toned stomach without moving a muscle—just buy this abs-sculpting electrical belt for 3 easy payments of $9.99!"

> "Need to lose weight? Simply sprinkle weight-loss crystals on your food, and you can eat as much as you want of all the foods you love!"

Do you think if I had just a handful of weeks to transform an actor's or athlete's body, my approach would be to have the person train his or her abs for 8 minutes a day and sprinkle fat-burning crystals on weight-loss cookies? Probably not. Yet people consistently fork over their hard-earned money for similar methods, believing they'll magically build a body like a movie star.

In 2012, the supplement industry was worth more than $32 billion. It's projected to grow to $60 billion[3] by 2021. The weight-loss market alone was worth $64 billion in 2014. With all the money spent on products to help people get fit and live healthier, you'd think that the majority of Americans would be walking around in incredible shape. Instead, the opposite is true—the National Institutes of Health reports[4] that about 70 percent of Americans are overweight. And research[5] shows that there are about 108 million dieters in the United States, and these people make four or five attempts at dieting each year.

Four or five attempts per year? How many times can a person go through that cycle of hope and ultimate failure before they just throw their hands up in the air and give up for good?

The cycle typically works like this: You see an ad for a product that promises big results, all in just a handful of weeks, with minimal effort on your part. So, you buy the product because, hey, why not? Plus, plastered on its label is some compelling, science-sounding jargon and a lot of great before-and-after photos. You use the product diligently. But when your handful of weeks are up, your results are far less impressive than promised, if you see any results at all.

How many times have you or someone you know been through this? Don't be ashamed if you have—numerous fitness products tricked me early in my career, and I don't know a single trainer who hasn't tried a method that promised big results that turned out to be less than effective. If you are a driven, committed, competitive person, you're probably always looking for an edge.

Bobby's Law:
Believe in yourself. You are capable of more than you think.

In this book, I'm not going to bullshit you. The truth is that there is no free lunch. There's no magic pill. You cannot get fit—and stay fit—on just three easy payments of $9.99, or on 10 minutes of exercise a day. Understand this: Becoming truly fit is never easy, nor should it be.

Most good things in life don't come easy. In fitness, the things that do come easy usually come with a catch—if a fat-loss or muscle-growth product really does work fast, it's probably illegal or will be soon. Reaching your goal always, always, always takes time and effort.

Consider this number: 1. That's the average number of hours per day of exercise that people who lost 30 pounds or more and kept it off for 5 years, according to the National Weight Control Registry.[6] That is far more than the standard 15 min-

utes a day, three times a week, that you're often told works.

Another number to consider: 94. That's the percent of those people who also improved their eating habits. For those people, none of that sustained weight loss happened through miracle diets. They haven't been sprinkling weight-loss crystals on their food for 5 years. Nearly 100 percent of them had to completely overhaul their diets.

After college, I found out just how much time it takes to reach a big goal, when I entered the world of kickboxing. Because I was already skilled at wrestling, I figured kickboxing would come easy. I began training in the sport four to five times a week, for about an hour each session. It wasn't always easy to make those sessions—I had a full-time job, and I also lived about 30 minutes away from the gym.

I progressed rather quickly and made improvements, but in all honesty, I really wasn't anything special. I was still a newcomer, and I made a lot of mistakes. After months of training, I entered my first few mixed martial arts and kickboxing fights. I had some decent fights, but the results weren't spectacular enough to put me on the radar of the big leagues. I was still a B-level fighter.

If I wanted to get where I wanted to be in the fight world, I needed to go all-in.

I decided to pack up all of my stuff and move. I rented a room in the same building on King Street in London, Ontario, where the fight gym was located. I literally lived in the same building I trained in.

That eliminated my commute, which gave me far more opportunities to train. In the morning, I would simply run downstairs and get to work. Instead of training four or five times a week, I started training two or three times a day. My life revolved around the sport. I trained in the morning, afternoon, and evening. When I wasn't in the gym, I watched film and studied.

Guess what happened? I became really good at kickboxing. Just 18 months after moving next to the gym, I fought for an International Kickboxing Federation world kickboxing championship. I won that fight, not because I was born with the innate ability to kickbox, but because I worked my ass off. Day in and day out, I put in the quality hours that I needed to succeed.

I'm not saying you need to live in the gym or train twice a day, but you do need to put in "quality hours." Even if you put in time, it can't be spent mindlessly going through the motions. It must be spent working, grinding, and feeling discomfort. Success is primarily a function of time and effort.

Put in that time and effort, and the real magic starts to happen. Once you learn to dedicate yourself and work hard, something occurs that I like to call a deep chemical change.

My friend Jason is the perfect example of this deep chemical change. Jason grew up in a small town in Oklahoma. He had a father who commuted 90 minutes each day so that he could raise his family in a small town and better teach them the values of old-fashioned hard work. Indeed, that was the greatest lesson Jason learned growing up.

Jason came from an athletic family. Two of his brothers were Division 1 NCAA athletes, and Jason played football in college. He graduated with a degree in chemical engineering.

After college, Jason traded the gym for his work desk, but he still ate like an active college football player. On the way from turning a $50,000 company into a $25-million-dollar company, Jason let his health go by the wayside. One day, he looked in the mirror and didn't recognize the man he'd turned into. He was 5'11" and 260 pounds, what most people would consider obese.

To find more time to focus on his health, he sold

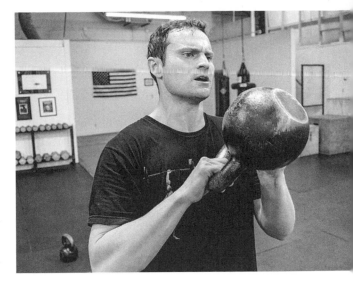

his business and took a new job as a vice president for another company. But that only made things worse—he was now on someone else's schedule, and it was a damned demanding schedule. His life was filled with stress, he was unable to do the things he loved, and he was unhappy. That was hurting his relationships with his family and causing him a deep sadness that he knew he needed to fix. He realized that he needed to change his entire life to be happy, and he started with his body.

Over the course of 6 months, he spent no less than 5 hours a week training. He regained his ability to do things like squat, deadlift, and row. The movements went from awkward to clean and smooth. Then, he added the strength he needed to put plates on his deadlift and squat, and the endurance he needed to row with vigor. Along the way, he lost 60 pounds.

With his weight loss, he gained something: A deep chemical change occurred within him.

The most important exercise Jason got out of training wasn't those deadlifts, squats, and rows. It was the confidence to take a short walk. One day, Jason strolled into his boss's office and put in his

Bobby's Law:
If the bar isn't bending,
there isn't enough weight on it.

2 weeks' notice, quitting the job he hated and deciding to move into investments so he could work at home, spend more time with his family, and do the things he loved.

You won't see a meaningful change by taking shortcuts. That kind of deep chemical change comes only from overcoming real challenges and putting in time and hard effort. Through failure, hard work, and then ultimately success in fitness, something happens to people. Psychologically, they become stronger. Building genuine fitness and horsepower and overcoming and facing fears in workouts transfers to every other area of life.

The confidence you get from rowing a sub-7-minute 2,000-meter row or deadlifting double body weight doesn't wash off with you in the shower. It stays with you, benefiting your every interaction thereafter.

No pill or easy payment can give you that. In fact, if there were a pill that would make me more fit than I am now, I wouldn't take it. Because no pill could ever replace the *real* benefit of reaching true fitness.

Doing things the right way isn't easy, but there are strategies that can help. These four tactics will help you hack your time management and also allow you to put forth more effort than you ever thought possible, helping you to reclaim your body and perform at your peak.

1. START SMALL, AND BUILD

It can be difficult to go from not training at all to carrying a full-time training schedule. I understand that all of a sudden adding 5 hours of training to your week can be stressful. Sure, I could lecture you about how you have to commit, but that wouldn't set you up for success. Instead, I'm just going to ask you to start small, and build from there.

Intensity is the inverse of duration. What I mean by that is that the harder you go—the more strict you go, the more extreme you go—the shorter the time you'll be able to sustain the effort. This is important because, in general, when the average person takes on a new fitness or eating plan, they tend to go from one end of the spectrum to the other. They go from eating whatever they want and sitting on the couch to jumping on a strict diet and into a grueling fitness plan.

What happens? Most of them last a month, if that. Then they burn out, quit, and go back to their old ways. We all know someone who's done this. Maybe you've even done this—I did early in my career.

Assuming that you're new or getting back into exercising and healthy eating, the problem is that going from an anything-goes way of life to a strict diet and exercise routine is like trying to drive a stick-shift when you only know how to ride a bike. Sure, you might manage for a time, but eventually you'll crash. The reason this approach fails isn't because you have shitty willpower or no commitment, it's because early into a fitness journey, you lack knowledge and can't handle the influx of changes.

Good habits can't be forced all at once. You have to build them over time. There is a certain type of personality who does well with a rush of extreme changes, but the vast majority of people will grasp and incorporate a few small changes at a time instead of everything all at once. Most important, this method will help those changes stay with you for the long haul.

If you're new to training and eating right, incorporate the dietary and training programs in this book into your day-to-day life slowly. Rather than overhauling every single thing you eat, try adopting one nutritional change every week. Instead of going from no exercise to adding a bunch of hours a week, your first couple weeks could be spent walking more and doing a few minutes a day of body-weight training. Then start with 1 day of gym training a week, and add from there every week until you are on the required schedule.

This may not seem like much at first, and you'll want to do more, but don't. Using this method, you'll ramp up to the nutritional guidelines and exercise programs in this book. You'll accumulate the habits you need to succeed in the long run.

If you already exercise and generally watch what you eat, jump right into the programs in this book. They might be a step up from what you're used to, but you can handle it—you already have a foundation of good habits to build upon.

2. SWEAT THE SMALL STUFF

People often think that fitness occurs only within the four walls of the gym. What you do in the gym is important, obviously, but it isn't the only thing that you can do to improve your fitness.

Bobby's Law:
You can never do too many pushups.

People assume that I spend all my time in a gym and use that to justify why I achieve my goals. But that's not necessarily true, nor has it always been the case. I've worked as a teacher, a police officer, and a business owner. I'm also a father, which is the most important responsibility I have—family always comes before fitness. But in all my roles, I've always found a way to train, regardless of whether or not I had extra time or access to a gym.

Take, for example, my approach to watching movies with my son. His two favorites are *The Lord of the Rings* and *The Hobbit*. If you have children,

you can name their favorite movies, and, chances are, like me, you've probably seen your kids' favorite movies a hundred times. I actually consider myself fortunate that I've only viewed the *The Lord of the Rings* and *The Hobbit* in the hundreds of times. If you're a dad with a young girl, you've probably seen *Frozen* just north of two thousand times.

When I watch *The Lord of the Rings* or *The Hobbit* (again) with my son, I could sit on the couch through the entire movie and do nothing, or I could throw in some exercise. I always choose the latter. Once, during a viewing of *The Hobbit*, I did 700 pushups. Another time, I did 1,000 body-weight squats. I talk to my son throughout, and it models good behavior for him. Sometimes, he'll even join me in a workout. Sure, it may not be the perfect workout, but the work is valuable, and by the end of the year (imagine how many TV shows or movies you watch in a year), the little bouts of hard work accumulate, and the results become apparent.

Doing this kind of small stuff is critical. If you miss the gym one day—or have time when you're watching TV or just hanging out—don't just do nothing. Accumulating small workouts, recovery practices (which you'll learn about soon), or other acts of fitness throughout the day, week, and month can have incredible long-term results.

For example, how many pushups do you think you've done in your life? One thousand? Five thousand? Ten thousand? Ten thousand seems like a lot of pushups, right? Try this: Do 5 pushups every half-hour for 10 hours out of each day (yes, you can do them in your office or other workplace). You'll never get tired or sweaty, and you'll never feel exhausted, but each day, you'll have accumulated 100 pushups. Do that for a year, and by the end of the year, you will have done more than 36,500 pushups. I think we can all agree that

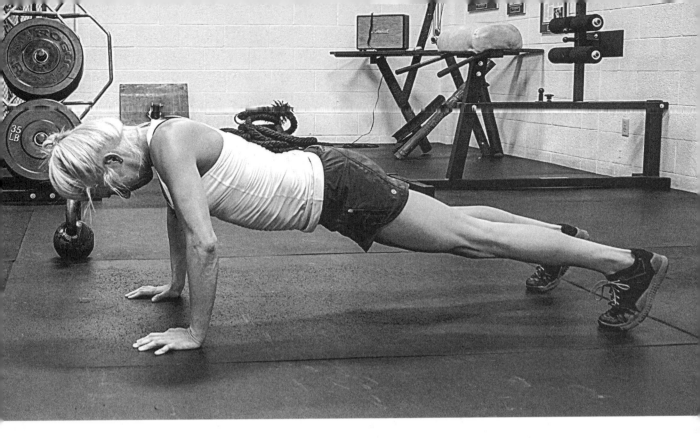

you'd be pretty damn strong if you did 36,500 pushups in a year.

Finding opportunities and striving to do the best you can in any situation will lead to incredible gains in your fitness. All you have to do is to get creative and consider every situation a potential chance for you to get closer to your goal.

3. EMBRACE THE MAXIMUS 130-HOUR RULE

For the majority of people, it takes roughly 130 quality hours to get fit. A lot of people ask me where I got that number. That number is the equivalent of training hard, an hour a day, 5 days a week, for 6 months.

If you're able to do that while paying attention to your behaviors outside of the gym (recovery and nutrition, which we'll talk about later), you'll be successful. Almost every single person that I've trained was able to make a radical transformation and see that deep chemical change—by way of an improved physique and excellent performance numbers in the gym—in 6 months' time following those parameters. Then, they only got better from there. One-hundred thirty hours in 6 months is the answer for most people, and it's totally doable.

Then again, people have made equally radical transformations in just 12 weeks—but the 130-hour rule still stands. If you want to get fit in 12 weeks, then training for just an hour a day, 5 days a week won't cut it—you'd only reach a total of 60 hours. That's nowhere near the 130 hours required to change. To accumulate 130 hours in 12 weeks, you'd have to train twice a day for an hour, Monday through Friday, and once on Saturday. That's a lot. But that's what it takes.

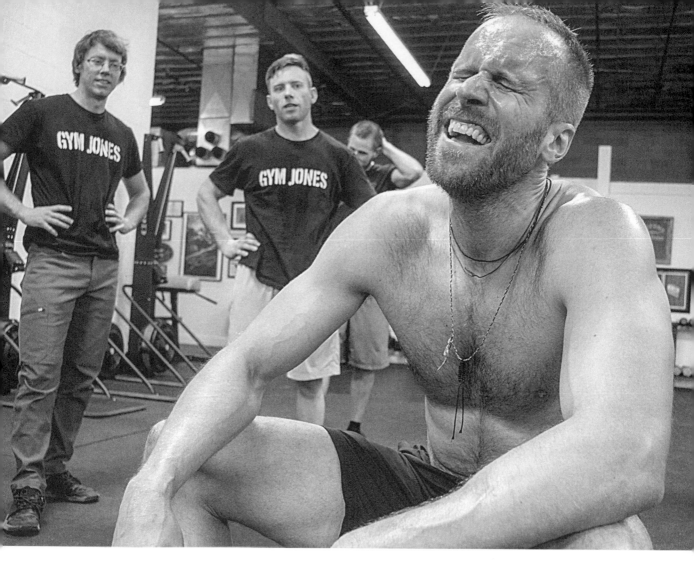

So, budget your time. Set your schedule however you want, but you can't cheat the end cost.

Think of this concept like taking a 15-year mortgage versus taking a 30-year mortgage. One gets you to the end goal faster, but it has much higher monthly payments. End of story. There's no shortcut or deal. The cost is the cost, and you cannot escape it: 130 hours is non-negotiable. There's no free lunch, shortcut, or time-saving technique here.

4. BUY IT ONCE

I used to be the king of buying $40 blenders. I don't know how many of them I've gone through in my life, but the number would alarm you. My blenders go through a whole hell of a lot of use. I drink a protein shake of some sort one or two times every day.

I remember standing at the store looking at all the options when I bought my first blender. The appliances ranged in price from $40 to $400.

Spending $400 on a blender seemed insane to me. What could it do that the $40 model couldn't? So, I grabbed the cheapest one and took it home. All blenders are the same right?

The unit blended just fine, but one morning, about 3 months later, it kicked mid-blend, and my kitchen filled with the tell-tale scent of a burned-out electrical motor. A blender doesn't last long in the world of Bobby Maximus.

I repeated this process for years. Then, one day, as I stood at the store staring at those blenders, something clicked. I was just so sick of replacing blenders that it occurred to me that maybe there was a difference between the $40 and $400 units.

So, I bought the $400 unit. I'd been through so many blenders at that point, I was willing to throw money at the problem.

When I unpacked it, I could see and feel the difference. It was heavier, more solid, and seemed to have the same horsepower as a compact car. The first time I used it, I was surprised at how fast it liquefied my meal.

I've had that damned blender for 4 years now, and it's now completed somewhere north of two thousand blends.

Because of that blender, I adopted a new rule, which I now understand applies to fitness: Buy it once. I would rather pay heavily up front and do things the right way the first time than have to constantly replace or fix things down the road.

The same basic rule applies to your own fitness—investing more time and effort early on results in long-lasting, quality fitness. Doing things the right way will ensure that you get the result that you are looking for.

If you decide to take the shortcut or easy way out, then your fitness simply won't last—if you even become fit in the first place. You'll keep trying new products, new programs, and fad diets, and you'll fail repeatedly. I've worked with many people who've experienced this. They spend years looking for the answer, searching for that one magic thing that will make all the difference. They jump from program to program and from product to product. Then, they work with me, put in the proper amount of work and effort, and discover that the secret was in front of their faces all those years: *hard work*.

If you dedicate real time and effort, you'll build a solid, sustainable foundation of genuine fitness that allows you to stay in shape in the long run.

Of course, you have to do consistent upkeep, and you should always try to improve. But the benefit of a strong foundation is this: When life happens—say, you hurt your knee skiing and can't do lower-body exercises for a couple months—you'll stay in greater shape and will be able to rebuild your fitness level faster.

That was the conclusion of Spanish scientists who looked at data on runners, rowers, and power athletes who took a month off from exercise. They found that once you build genuine strength, your body tries to hold on to that strength for as long as it possibly can.

I did it the right way, the harder way. I spent the time up front and never looked for a shortcut. Because of that, I have been able to remain fit for more than 20 years. Even if I took a year off, I would still be more fit than the vast majority of people. Why? I've laid the right foundation. I make every single person I work with do it the right way, too, so their fitness lasts.

I want the same for you. Now, let's learn how to do just that.

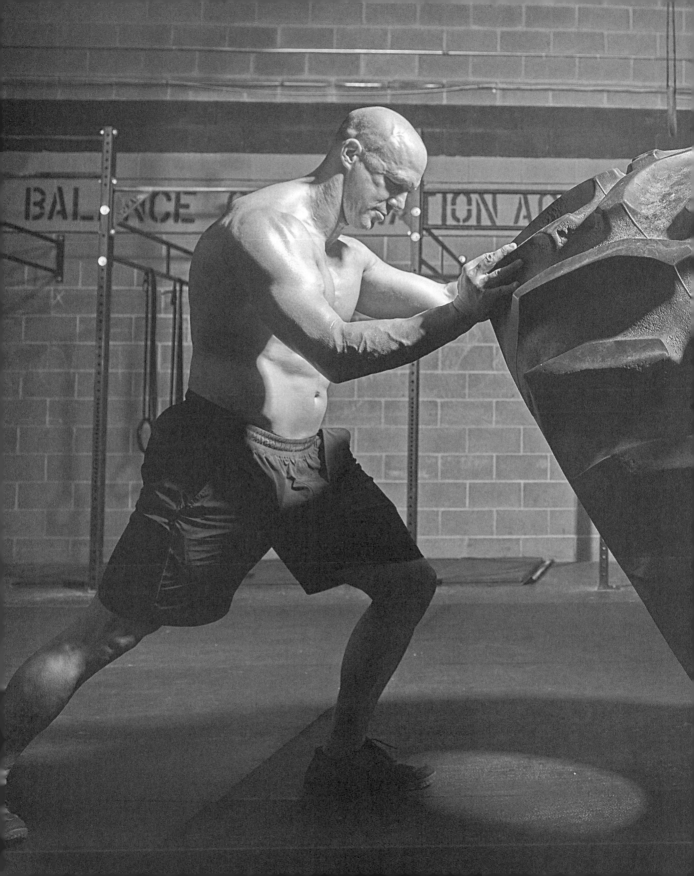

TRAINING

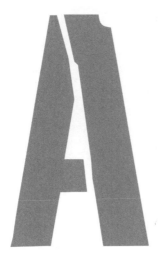

A successful training method has two components: working smart and working hard.

You could have the most brilliantly designed fitness plan in the world, but if you don't do it intensely, it'll take you nowhere. Conversely, if you work your ass off doing the wrong things, you'll only end up somewhere you don't want to be or on the injured list.

Today, most training programs fail not because they lack one of these components, but because they lack both of them—they're designed to be as simplistic and effortless as possible.

Look at anyone who has accomplished an important physical goal, whether it's doing something like running a marathon in less than 3 hours or losing 100 pounds.

They had to develop carefully considered plans. They had to then follow those plans diligently and put in an incredible amount of hard work and effort. The process surely wasn't quick or easy, but I guarantee that in both of these examples, the people would say that it was highly worth it. Self-improvement is always worth it.

In this section, you'll learn to work both smarter *and* harder. You'll first learn the single-most important decision you can make before you even set foot in the gym. Then, you'll learn exactly what you should do once you're ready to tackle a training program. The methods featured in this section aren't the easiest, but they also make each moment that you spend working out that much more effective. Next, you'll find out exactly what your training plan should focus on so that you can not only reach your goal but also perform well in any task that life throws at you. Finally, you'll learn about a biological phenomenon that, at this very moment, is preventing you from giving exercise your all, thereby holding you back. I'll show you a technique to overcome it, so you can work harder and achieve a level of fitness that you never thought possible.

The end result is that you'll master exactly how to work the right way, and you'll be able to tackle anything you want with confidence. A new you awaits . . .

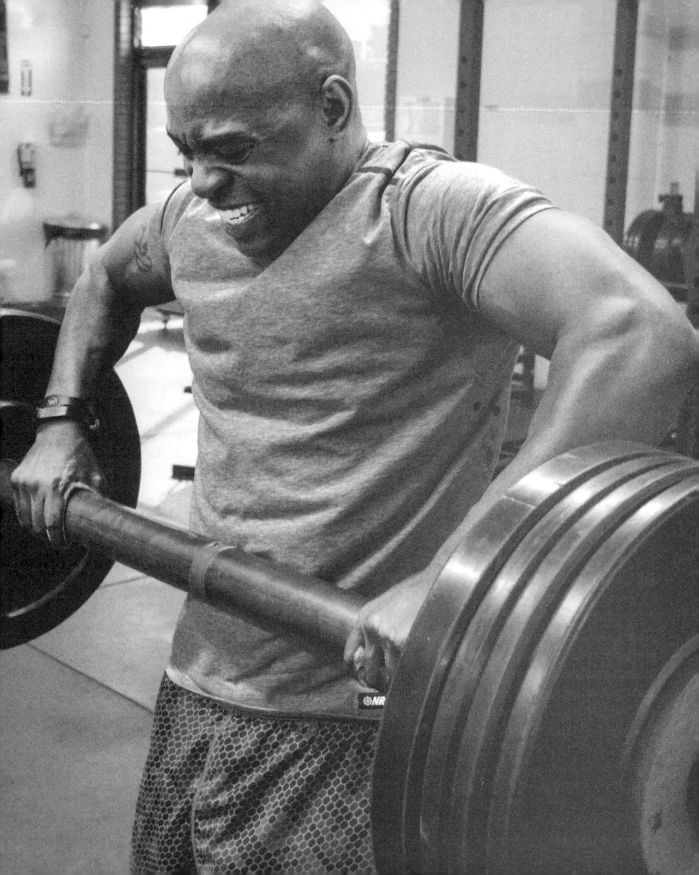

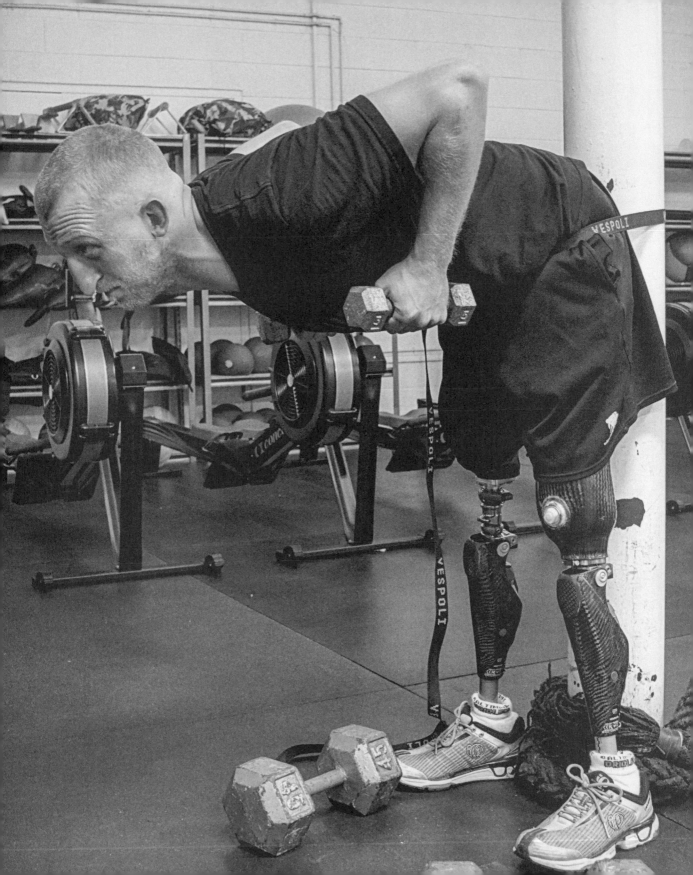

5

SET A GOAL

In 2007, my friend Rob Jones joined the Marine Corps Reserves as a combat engineer. He specialized in explosives and detecting buried improvised explosive devices.

Rob first deployed to Habbaniya, Iraq, in 2008, then was sent to Sangin, Afghanistan, in 2010. During that last deployment, he was part of an operation that pushed deep into Taliban territory. One day, Rob was sent to clear an area that the marines believed might be filled with improvised explosives. It was. As he worked, one tripped. The blast took both of Rob's legs just above his knee area.

After emergency surgery in Afghanistan, Rob was flown back to the United States to be fitted for prosthetics and to begin rehabilitation. The nurses told him that he had to learn to walk again, an infinitely harder task when your amputation is above the knee joint.

It wasn't easy, but he did it. Once he accomplished his goal of being able to put one foot in front of the other on his own, he set another pivotal goal: to bring home a medal in the mixed double scull rowing event in the 2012 Paralympics in London. The United States had never medaled in that event before.

The fact that Rob had never rowed mattered little to him. He simply believed that if he worked hard enough, he'd bring that medal to American soil.

Rob was well aware that extreme goals take extreme measures. So he dedicated himself fully. He and his partner, Oksana Masters, immediately moved to Florida, because it was the perfect place to train for the mixed-double scull event—an event where one man and one woman row together. The two spent time in Florida, winning various trunk and arms double-scull trials races held by US Rowing, which made them the US Rowing national team for their boat class. Next, they won the final Paralympic qualification regatta, in Belgrade, qualifying them for the Paralympic games.

Then, Rob's training only intensified. He and Oksana moved to Charlottesville, Virginia, and trained together twice a day nearly every single day of the week. Some sessions they might row for 2 hours straight to build their aerobic capacity, other sessions they'd do 90-minute weight circuits. When he wasn't in the boat or at the gym, he was eating healthy to fuel his training, or he was sleeping or doing other recovery practices to stay refreshed and injury-free.

Because of all that hard work and constant attention to his goal, Rob felt confident when he landed in London. He and his partner performed strong in the initial heats. Once they hit the finals, their hard work paid off: Rob and Oksana landed on the podium by beating out a British boat by less than a second.

Rob didn't stop there. Once he had his medal, he decided to set another goal: to ride his bike across the country to raise more than $125,000 for military veteran charities. His journey took him 181 days and 5,180 miles from Bar Harbor, Maine, to Camp Pendleton, California. It surely wasn't easy—because he had prosthetics from the thigh down, he had less muscle to put into each pedal stroke—but he put his head down, focused on the goal, and made it.

Each of Rob's journeys changed his life for the better and, more important, allowed him to inspire other people, especially wounded veterans. Rob didn't have an advantage over anyone else. He

Bobby's Law:
Keep your head high and your middle finger higher.

wasn't lucky. In fact, you could argue that he was at a disadvantage and was unlucky. But he was able to do great things because he set a firm goal and then let that goal guide every single thing he did thereafter.

Spinning your wheels gets you nowhere—to reach real fitness and have your training create a deep chemical change, you need to start with a goal. Your goals don't have to be as grand as Rob's, but clear goals are necessary for progress.

The benefit of goal-setting is twofold. First, you'll see more benefits from your training. You'll no longer be able to just pick exercises and workouts at random. You'll need to follow a structured fitness plan, which helps you make more significant improvements. It also often puts you on a deadline.

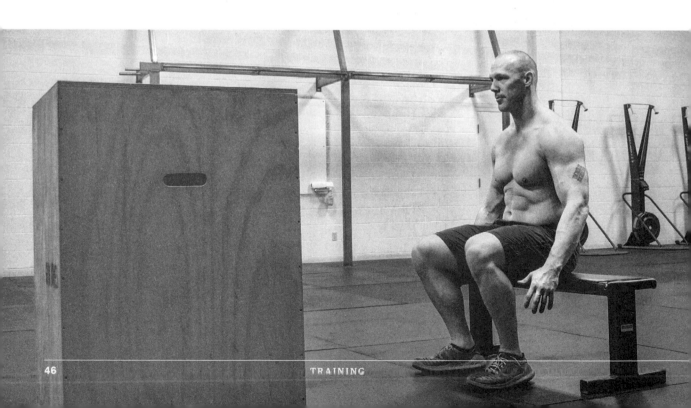

That makes each workout critical, so you'll consistently exercise, which is the key to improvement.

Second, having a goal gives meaning to your training. Along the way, you'll have setbacks relative to your goal, you'll rise above them, and then you'll become mentally and physically stronger compared to how you were on day one. Through this process, you'll experience that deep chemical change, helping you become a completely improved person.

But setting a goal isn't quite as simple as declaring that you want to do something. When I first meet a new trainee, we go over these seven guidelines designed to help them find a life-changing goal, and stick to it so they can see incredible change.

1. NAME YOUR GOAL

Sit down and think about what's truly important to you. What single thing might change your life? For most people, it's to lose weight, build more strength or muscle, or accomplish something like a triathlon, mountain climb, or backcountry hunting or skiing trip. Dream big: I think anyone with enough dedication can lose any amount of weight, put on up to 20 or even 30 pounds of muscle, and finish any life-altering race or climb.

2. ANALYZE YOUR GOAL

Now that you have an objective, figure out what fitness skills you'll need to achieve it. This is straightforward for some goals, like marathoning or powerlifting. But for others, it can be confusing. If you want to lose weight or gain muscle, food plays a large role, so you'll have to consider your needs in the kitchen as well as in the gym. Many sports, like

mountain climbing, triathlons, hunting, and skiing, require strength, power, and endurance, as well as a high level of technical skill, so you'll need to improve yourself across the board.

3. TEST YOURSELF

Now that you have an objective, you need to figure out where you are in relation to your objective. So, test yourself. If you want to run a marathon, for example, you might go out and see how quickly you can run 5 miles. If you want to put 50 pounds on a lift, see how strong you are right now. For goals like losing weight or gaining muscle, have your body composition tested. If your goal was to complete a hunting trip, you might test your endurance by backpacking, and also your shooting accuracy. No matter your goal, test yourself in a handful of fitness tests, like those in the "May I Suggest a Goal?" box on page 48. Whether you're trying to look or perform better, improving the skills you're lacking helps propel you closer to your goal. If you have a strength goal but the tests, for example, reveal that you are seriously lacking endurance, improving your endurance may allow you to gain strength by helping you pump blood more efficiently and recover quicker.

4. FIND A TRAINING PLAN

Once you know where you want to be (goal) and how you need to get there (based on your analysis and tests), find a plan that fits. If your goal is to lose weight, build muscle, or build elite fitness, you can follow the programs in this book and tweak your nutrition appropriately. For other goals, you can string together the workouts in this book to create a plan that will help you reach your goal. If your goal is to build strength, for example, you might perform the strength month (see "Block 3: Weeks 9 to 12" on page 125) from the The 6-Month Program.

5. EXECUTE YOUR PROGRAM

This is the easy part: Show up and work hard. Take notes as you go through the first 4 to 8 weeks of your program about what exercises feel hardest, where you think you need to improve, where you're improving, and anything else you think is relevant.

6. RETEST, ANALYZE YOUR RESULTS, AND RETHINK

After 4 to 8 weeks of training, retest yourself. If you're headed in the right direction, continue to work hard and don't change anything. If things aren't improving, analyze what's holding you back. Are you not working hard enough? Are you not eating appropriately? Is it recovery? Once you think you have the answer, make the appropriate tweak.

7. KEEP EXECUTING

Simply continue to work hard in the gym, retest yourself, and revise continually until you reach your goal.

This process takes more work, consideration, and dedication than simply exercising at random and hoping it'll get you to your goal. But it's also the right way. By investing up front, you'll accomplish more and save yourself time and headaches along the way.

MAY I SUGGEST A GOAL?

Having trouble finding a goal? How about working toward hitting all 20 of these fitness standards? It doesn't matter if you weigh 125 pounds or 250 pounds. If you can reach and maintain them all, you're a person who can lift heavy and go for long durations—and can ultimately handle anything physical life throws at you. These tests can also give you a sense of what skills you're "good" at, and which you need to improve. If, for example, you find you can hit all of the strength standards but fail most cardio-based standards, make sure that your program favors more cardio over weight lifting.

Back squat: 2 times your body weight	1,000-meter row: 3:30
Deadlift: 2.5 times your body weight	1,000-meter ski: 3:30
Front squat: 1.5 times your body weight	2,000-meter row: 7:00
Overhead squat: 1.25 times your body weight	2,000-meter ski: 7:00
Bench press: your body weight for 10 reps	5,000-meter row: 18:30
Power clean: 1.25 times your body weight	5,000-meter ski: 18:30
Turkish getup: half your body weight	1.5-mile run: 8:45
500-meter row: 1:30	60-minute row: 15,400 meters
500-meter ski machine: 1:30	60-minute ski: 15,400 meters
60-second fan bike: 55 calories	10K run: 50 minutes

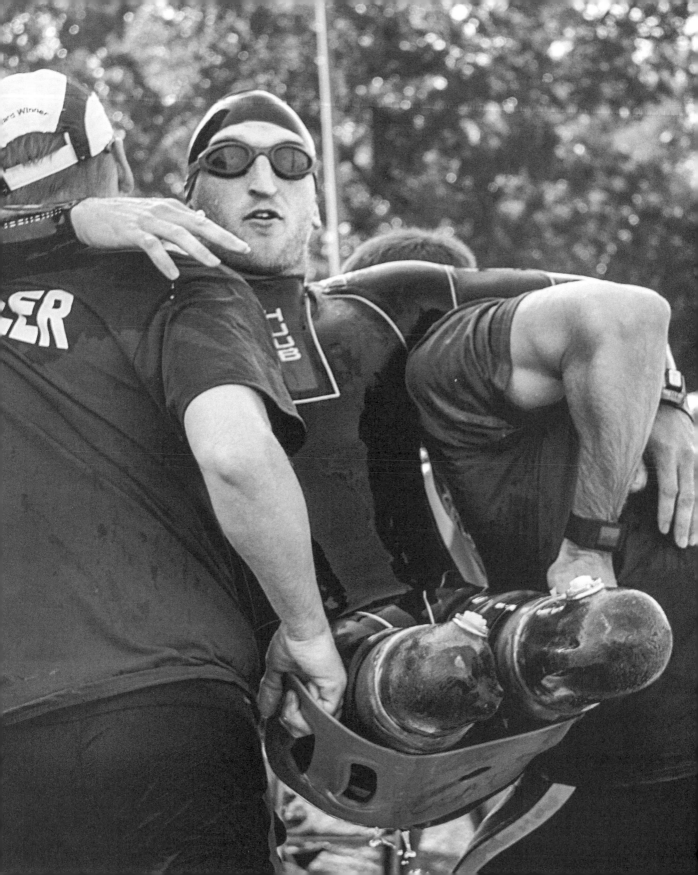

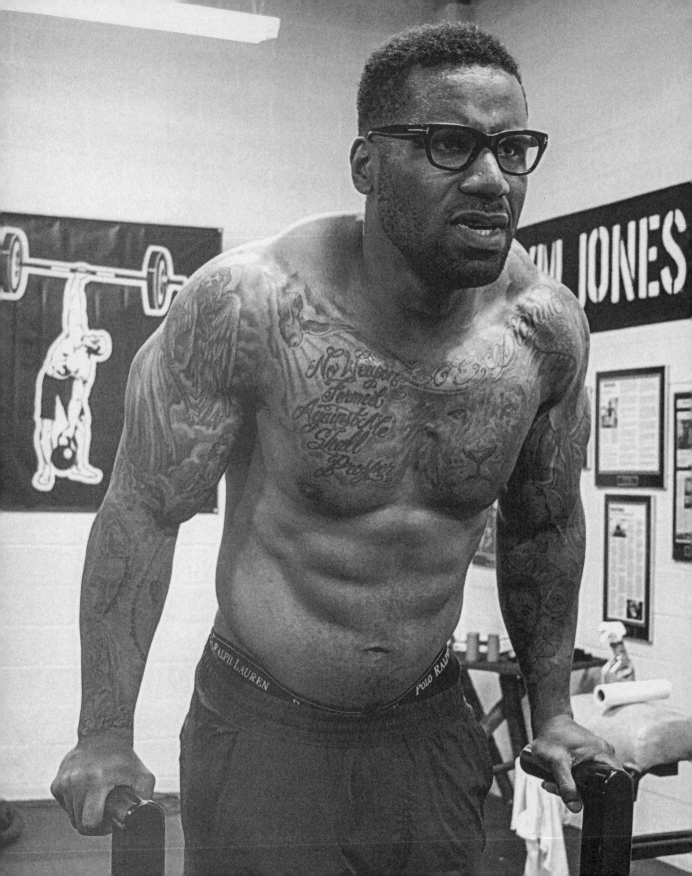

6

TRAIN FOR LIFE

If you go into the average big-box gym, you'll find machines: biceps curl machines, chest press machines, chest fly machines, leg press machines, leg extension machines, ab crunch machines, triceps press-down machines. The list goes on and on—if you have a muscle you want to work, the average gym has multiple machines that you can work it with.

In many of those big-box gyms, free weights like dumbbells and barbells are relegated to a small corner of the gym, if they exist at all. Why do gyms do this?

It's simple: Machines require little instruction, so the gym doesn't have to teach you how to exercise. You just look at the little illustration slapped on the side of the machine, and follow along. These devices also make the gym seem special, like you're buying into something that you could never replicate at home. The average person, for example, could spend a few hundred dollars and fill his garage with dumbbells and work his entire body with them. But it would take thousands of dollars to fill your garage with enough machines to work your entire body.

Not all machine exercises are bad, but most

are less than ideal. That's because you perform most of those exercises sitting down, with your limbs stabilized, on a fixed range of motion. Take machine biceps curls, for example. You select a weight, take a seat, place your elbows against a pad, grab some ergonomic handles, then move those handles up and down a fixed track, moving just your forearms and hands. When do you ever perform a movement like that in the real world? Here's how those four aspects of machine training set you up for failure.

▶ **You Sit Down**
Sport and everyday physical tasks are rarely performed sitting down. So exercising in the sitting position doesn't prepare your body for any actual event, whether it's something like running or just playing with your kids. Sure, in sports like cycling or rowing, you sit, but your upper and lower body both move heavily throughout those sports. In machine exercises, your upper or lower half is typically static. What's more, you probably sit too much at work already. The Mayo Clinic reports that sitting for 10 hours each day (that sounds like

a lot, but it's the national average) cancels out 90 percent of a 60-minute workout. Most alarming, the Mayo Clinic also says that sitting excessively can negatively affect your life expectancy.[1]

▶ **You Stabilize Your Joints**

When you do a machine exercise, the body part that you're working is usually stabilized against a pad. In the biceps curl, for example, your upper arms are on a pad; in an overhead press, your shoulders are against a pad; in a leg extension, your upper leg is resting on a pad. If you were doing similar movements in the real world, you wouldn't have this source of stability. When you move an object (or free weight like a dumbbell, barbell, or kettlebell) through open air, you have to find stability from small stabilizing muscles throughout your body, and in your core. Machines take these muscles out of the equation, which also causes you to work less muscle overall, making each rep less effective. It's also dangerous in the long run: While machines make the muscle you're trying to work strong, your stabilizing muscles stay weak. Then, when you go out and move in the real world, your primary muscles can overpower your stabilizing muscles, causing injury.

▶ **You Move through a Fixed Range of Motion**

Machine exercises all run on a track. Your muscles make the same, shortened movement every single rep. Not moving your muscle through a full range of motion leads to stiffness and makes each rep less effective, simply because you're moving a weight over less distance. And in the real world, your body moves in all different planes: forward, backward, side-to-side, diagonal. If you only go one direction, as machines have you do, you'll limit your ability to move in those other planes of motion, which is key for all sports and for living and moving in the real world.

▶ **You Isolate Your Muscles**

The majority of machines are designed to train a muscle group in isolation. But your brain doesn't think in terms of working muscles. It only knows movements: primarily the squat, hip hinge, push, pull, and plank. By forcing you to isolate muscles with mechanized, unrealistic movements, your muscles work less cohesively together, decreasing your performance. That isolation can also cause strength imbalances and problems in your connective tissues, which can set you up for injury.

The big-picture knock on machines: They make you strong in a way that not only doesn't transfer to the real world, they also potentially set you up for problems and injuries.

Bobby's Law:

Above all else, you have to want it.

So what should you do? Free-weight exercises. The majority of free-weight exercises force you to engage your entire body—including your stabilizing muscles—and move athletically, and also challenge your balance, coordination, and range of motion.

Some of my favorite exercises of all time include squats, deadlifts, presses, burpees, dips, pullups, and pushups. Yes, they feel more intense than the average machine move. But that's because you're working more muscle, and working it harder—which means you'll see more bang for your buck for each rep and reach your physique goals faster.

Each of those exercises falls into one of the five aforementioned basic human movement patterns, which are: the squat (bending at your knees and hips), hip hinge (bending at your hips), push (pushing something away from you), pull (pulling something toward you), and plank (keeping your torso stiff). You see those five movements in nearly anything you do.

Those kinds of exercises transfer over to any goal that you're aiming for and will make you perform better, whether you're playing pickup basketball, hiking, or just picking your kid up from the ground. Even the cardio machines I recommend you use—the fan bike, rowing machine, treadmill, and ski ergometer—require that you use your entire body as a cohesive unit.

Consider, for example, if you were training to climb Mount Kilimanjaro. Doing a bunch of leg extensions while sitting down on a leg extension machine doesn't look like any movement you'd perform while climbing that peak. Doing weighted lunges and stepups, some loaded carries, and squats, on the other hand, would transfer well and help you accomplish your goal.

You see the movements in ball sports, too. Consider the job of J. J. Watt, arguably the best defensive player in the National Football League. Before a play starts, he assumes a slight lunge position (squat), with his hips back (hinge). The opposing quarterback yells "hike," and J. J. explodes from his

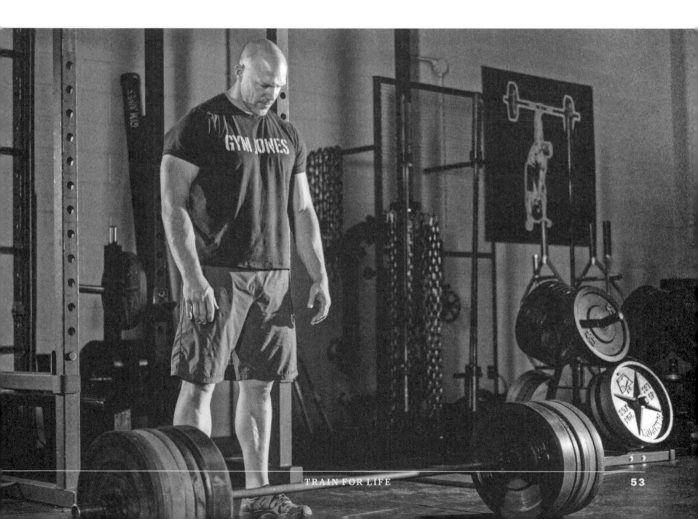

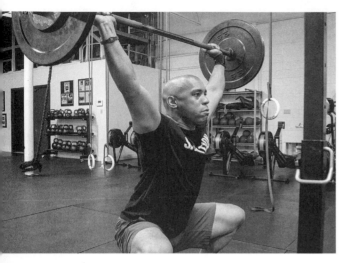

hips (hinge) to sprint forward. Along the way, he'll bash into the offensive lineman and bull him out of the way (push), or rip him to the ground (pull). Once he reaches the quarterback, he'll quickly push his hips back (hinge) and then explode forward, straightening his body (plank) as he tackles the quarterback.

The guy who climbs Kilimanjaro and J. J. are both incredible athletes and seemingly different athletes, but they perform the exact same movements—even you do the same basic movements every day. You bend down to pick things up (hinge), get in and out of the car or a chair (squat), and carry things (plank). Moving through life is one big series of pushing, pulling, hinging, squatting, and planking movements.

That's why selecting the right exercises for the climber, J. J. Watt, you, or anyone else is actually the easy part: Grab some free weights and do exercises that take you through basic movements. I've found that everyone from beginners to pros sees the biggest benefits from just a handful of basic exercises. In fact, one of the primary reasons professionals are so good at what they do is that they are absolute masters of the basics.

Where you, the climber, and J. J. Watt may also differ is in how many sets and reps you do, at what speed you do the reps, how long your rest periods are, and, of course, how much weight you use.

Once you've incorporated free-weight exercises that focus on working movements over individual muscles, it's time to consider how you should build your body.

I can't begin to count the number of men I've worked with who want to look like The Rock, but because Utah—where I live—is an outdoor sports Mecca, they also want to perform at a high level in endurance sports like ski mountaineering, rock climbing, mountain biking, or cross-country skiing. I tell them this: Pick one or the other. If you look like The Rock, you can't be elite in endurance events. If you're elite in endurance events, you can't look like The Rock. (You'll learn more about why in the next chapter.)

To illustrate how your body type can either make or break your performance, I use this analogy: If you had a 300-horsepower engine and needed to drive across the country as fast as possible, would you put that engine in a big, heavy truck, or in a small, light car? If you put it in the truck, your engine will have to work harder to push the big vehicle forward, costing you more gas and slowing you down. In the smaller, lighter car, you'll be able to go farther for each gallon of gas, and also faster.

But if you needed to, say, tow something, you'd probably want the truck. Its bigger, stronger frame could better bear the load. Trying to pull something big with the car's small, light frame would likely just warp it.

The point is this: Certain body types are conducive to certain goals. If your goal, like mine, is to be big and strong, that's great. Being bigger and stronger typically improves your performance in sports where short bursts of power are key. If you need to

LIFTING CAN HELP YOUR ENDURANCE

An incredible number of studies prove lifting weights can make you a better endurance athlete. In a 12-week study in the *British Journal of Sports Medicine*, scientists had one group of people run, one group lift, and one group both run and lift. The scientists found that, compared to the people who only ran or lifted, the group who combined strength and endurance training ran the fastest 4K race, and also could run 13.7 percent longer before becoming exhausted.[2]

Another study conducted by researchers in Norway found that seasoned runners who did barbell squats a few days a week for 8 weeks improved their endurance at maximum speed by 21 percent.[3] That can be a game changer if you're trying to pull ahead of someone close to the finish line.

The benefits of strength training extend to nearly all endurance sports. Cyclists who lifted saw a boost in their cycling economy, endurance, and power, according to a study in the *Journal of Strength and Conditioning Research*.[4]

move some serious weight to reach your goal or succeed in your sport—whether that weight is in the form of a defensive lineman or a loaded barbell—bigger is often better. Bigger frames can usually give and take a hit and move more weight. But that size also comes with a cost: You're bad over the long haul.

Bobby's Law:
It doesn't matter how you start. It matters how you finish.

In any sports where you have to carry your engine—move your body across a long distance—you want to be powerful but keep your weight as low as possible. If you plan on running long distances often, for example, being heavier—even if the weight is from muscle—is only going to slow you down and lead to greater impact on your joints with every step. Mountain climbers, for example, obsess over every ounce of gear they carry and often spend hundreds more dollars on a piece of equipment that's just a handful of ounces lighter. Any extra weight requires more effort for every

foot they climb. That's why they also try to keep their body weights as low as possible, while maintaining their strength.

If your goal is general fitness, to be someone who's relatively good in both endurance and strength, you'll want a body type somewhere between an ultralight marathoner and super-size strongman. In the car world, you'd put that 300-horsepower engine in something like a small or midsize SUV. It'd be light and streamlined enough that you'd still see decent gas mileage, but also burly enough that you can move some weight. Of course, you'd never beat our big guy in a strength competition, or our light guy in a marathon, but you could perform respectably in both.

CrossFit Games competitors are probably the ultimate showcase of this good-at-everything body type, and the winning males typically weigh around 190 pounds. But even these elite athletes aren't beating a real marathoner or strongman at their sport.

The lesson: Analyze your goal and its requirements. Then, build your program—and your body—based on your findings.

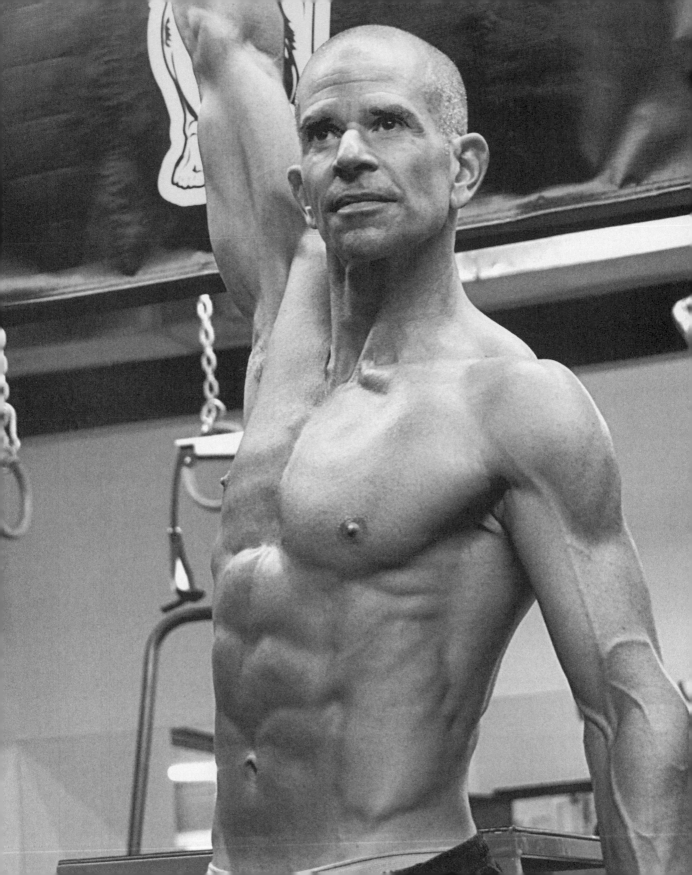

BE GOOD AT EVERYTHING

Paul Timmons, a 47-year-old gym owner from Rehoboth Beach, Delaware, is one of the very first people that I gave full instructor certification to at Gym Jones. With his bald head, small stature, and glasses, he looks rather unassuming. If you had to guess what he does for a living, you might peg him for a high-school math teacher, or maybe an accountant. That's why most people are shocked when I mention that he's actually one of the fittest men to ever train with me or at Gym Jones.

In fact, if you were to hold a fitness competition where competitors had to lift and then run a long distance, I'd put money on Paul to win. The guy set a Delaware State Powerlifting record when he deadlifted 485 pounds at a body weight of just 164 pounds. He also completed three Ironman competitions in Kona—2.4-mile swim, 112-mile bike ride, 26.2-mile run—and his best time is 11 hours.

Recently, Paul was the top-placing American in the CRASH-BB Indoor Rowing World Championships, finishing a 2,000-meter row in 6:45 in the Men's Lightweight 40–49 category.

Paul is a living example of a fitness principle that I've always preached: Train to be good at any physical task life throws at you.

There are many people today who choose only one fitness skill to train at the expense of all others. Marathoners fall into the trap of only running, lifters choose to only lift, and bodybuilders decide to only build muscle.

But a person who trains—and excels—in both endurance and strength is someone who has truly usable fitness. What's the point of being able to deadlift a compact car if you become winded walking up a flight of stairs? Who cares if you can run a fast marathon if you don't have the strength to pick up your kid and carry her when she becomes too tired to walk on a family vacation? My personal goal has always been to be the "big guy," but I've also made it clear that there's no use in being big if I can't move well and cover ground quickly.

There are two reasons people neglect to train other fitness skills. First, they don't realize that exercising in other ways will actually make them better at their primary sport (more on that soon). Second, they believe in the idea of "specialization."

Specialization in fitness is the idea that all fitness skills have a cost, and to improve in one skill, such as running, you must become worse in another, such as strength. Proponents of specialization point to marathoners and powerlifters as primary examples of why you should specialize.

Running marathons and powerlifting require completely opposite skills. The former requires a robust cardiovascular system and well-trained slow-twitch muscle fibers, which are muscle fibers built to power lower-intensity, long-duration activities like running, walking, or cycling. Those fibers are extremely efficient at doing low-power activities for a long amount of time. Think of them as the Toyota Prius of muscle fibers—they can go a long distance on just a little bit of fuel.

Powerlifting, on the other hand, requires you to use and build your fast-twitch muscle fibers. These fibers are designed to drive short, powerful efforts, such as lifting something heavy a couple of times, or sprinting a short distance, like 100 meters. They have little endurance, require a lot of fuel, but move big weights and propel you from point A to point B very quickly. That's why I like to think of them as the drag racers—hugely powerful for just a handful of seconds but inefficient over the long haul.

Proponents of specialization argue that when a marathoner starts to lift heavy, he decreases his efficiency. That's because strength training adds size to all of his muscle fibers, making him stronger, yes, but also hurting his ultimate goal of running 26.2 miles as fast as possible. It's like throwing a bunch of heavy luggage on top of your Prius. You now have to carry that extra weight, and the miles per gallon you see from your tank drops. You can either slow down to

THE TWO BIG FITNESS SKILLS
There are two very basic categories that go into overall fitness.

STRENGTH AND POWER

Power is moving something fast—all-out or close to all-out efforts. Strength is slow and grinding, like a deadlift, squat, or bench press. Power is fast and explosive, like a box jump or 40-yard dash. These efforts tax your fast-twitch muscle fibers, which are designed for short, intense efforts.

CARDIOVASCULAR FITNESS

Cardiovascular fitness is the ability of your heart and lungs to supply oxygenated blood to your muscles, and the ability of your muscles to use that oxygen to create energy. In basic terms: It's your body's ability to breathe, process oxygen, and go hard over a longer period of time without becoming too tired. In the realm of cardiovascular fitness, there exist two subcategories: power endurance and endurance. Power endurance is your body's ability to go hard at less than 100-percent effort for a moderate period of time, anywhere from 30 seconds to upward of 2 hours. Workouts that tax this system are the 1.5-mile run or the 2,000-meter row. Endurance, on the other hand, is your ability to move at a consistent pace for 3 hours or more. Endurance events are longer, lower-intensity efforts—events like marathon running or mountain climbing.

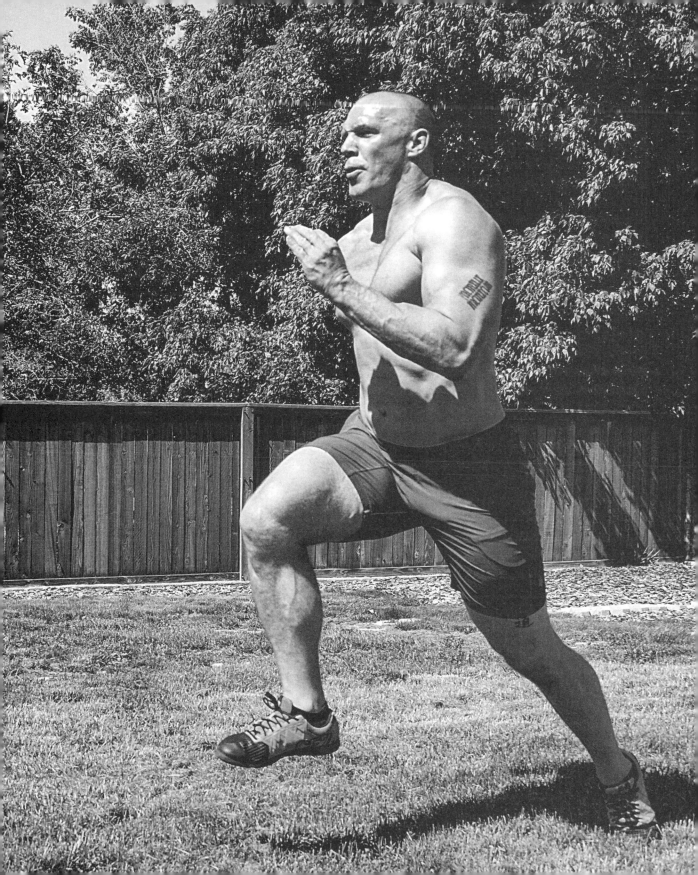

Be the person you want to be around.

maintain efficiency or run out of gas before you reach the finish line.

The equivalent argument for powerlifters is that when a powerlifter starts to do cardiovascular exercise, he replaces some of his powerful fast-twitch fibers for the slow-twitch variety. The powerlifter may now have more endurance, but it's at the expense of his strength. It's like downgrading the engine of your drag racer in order to drive it farther and save on gas mileage. That puts him at a disad-

vantage when he's trying to generate as much power as possible for a big lift.

Here's the problem: This argument only holds true at the highest levels of elite sports. This means, yes, that a marathon runner who runs a marathon around a 5-minute-mile pace probably shouldn't try to gain too much strength, or else his speed and endurance will drop, and a powerlifter who can deadlift more than 1,000 pounds likely shouldn't go out for long runs, or he'll lose some strength.

When I teach seminars or help people with their goals, there are inevitably those who think that they should specialize, because they'd like to be just as

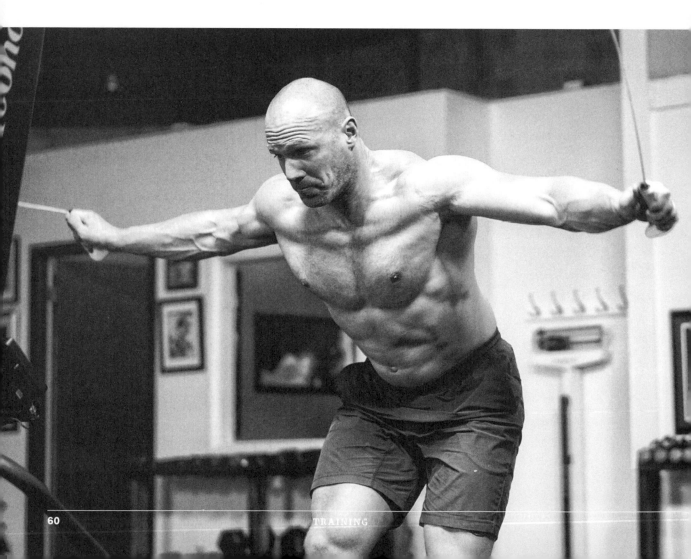

TRAINING

HEALTH BENEFITS OF STRENGTH TRAINING

Whether you care about performance or you're just training for general health, lifting is essential. It helps you:

- **Forge strong bones.** This reduces your risk of fracture and osteoarthritis.
- **Maintain a healthy weight.** Lifting boosts your resting metabolism, so you burn more calories after your workout. That higher metabolism makes it easier to keep your weight in check.
- **Boost your balance.** This makes you less likely to get hurt when you're off-balance in activities you enjoy (such as trail running), and also reduces your risk of falling around the house, which is key to preventing injury as you age.
- **Improve your quality of life.** Because it helps make physical activities easier—playing with your kids, carrying groceries, hiking, golfing—you'll enjoy yourself more.
- **Manage chronic conditions.** Strength training has been shown to help reduce your risk and symptoms of diabetes, heart disease, depression, arthritis, and general pain.
- **Build a better brain.** Some research suggests that lifting can improve your thinking and learning skills.[5]

good as the best in the world. I'm sorry, but for the average person, that's not realistic. It takes years of round-the-clock training to reach that level. You essentially have to become a full-time athlete and do nothing else. There is also a catch to specialization: It makes you worse at everything else. With world-class skill in one area of fitness comes a deficiency in other fitness skills, not to mention a host of sport-induced imbalances and health issues.

Don't get me wrong, I think specialization is great for a person who is winning championships, competing as a professional, or earning a living from his or her sport. But how many people do you know who are in that boat? How many people do you know that can run a sub-2:15 marathon or deadlift more than 1,000 pounds? The average person is not even close to the highest, elite level of their favorite activity.

So what should you do? No matter your goal, train like someone who wants to be good at everything. With that approach, you can build an incredible level of real-world fitness that improves your overall health and abilities.

You won't be giving up anything with that approach. Here's why: Most people can develop all

of their fitness skills at the same time to a level that's around 70 percent of their full biological capacity.

Of course, once you reach 70 percent of your full biological capacity, becoming better in one skill requires that others become worse. Paul, for example, is probably at his limit for strength and cardiovascular fitness. If he wants to do both at once, he won't be able to improve in one without the other suffering. If Paul wanted to deadlift 550 pounds, for example, he'd likely have to let his Ironman time slide to 12 hours. If he wanted to finish that Ironman in 10 hours, he'd probably have to let his deadlift drop to 435 pounds.

But the reality is that hitting 70 percent of your capacity in just one fitness skill is remarkable for the average person—it's incredibly strong or fast. So, first shoot to reach that level across the board. If you can do that, you'll be like Paul. He's fitter than 99.9 percent of the population, which is an incredible accomplishment.

This approach also makes your life more enjoyable. If you're a person who does a lot of activities with friends, it means that you can sign up for a 10K at the last minute and place well, then the next

HEALTH BENEFITS OF CARDIOVASCULAR ACTIVITY

Perhaps the biggest reason I tell people I train to do endurance work is that it's incredibly beneficial for your health. Doing cardiovascular activity can help you:

- **Avoid heart disease.** Heart disease is the number-one killer of American men and women. Cardio exercise helps your heart pump blood more efficiently and improves your heart health.
- **Ward off other chronic conditions.** Your risk of diabetes, depression, cancer, metabolic syndrome, and high cholesterol drops if you do aerobic exercise regularly.
- **Stay illness-free.** It can improve your immune system, so you'll be better able to escape the common cold.
- **Be happy.** Cardio exercise is linked to improved mood: It releases feel-good chemicals, like endorphins, and decreases chemicals linked to depression.

weekend do something like a Spartan Race, all the while lifting in the gym in the middle of the week. If you decide to try a new sport or activity, having a base of all-around fitness makes you far more likely to perform well and enjoy yourself.

Take me, for example. Even though my goal is to be the biggest, strongest guy at any gym I walk into, I do plenty of cardiovascular work every week and can run a 10K in 50 minutes. It's not only helped me reach my primary goal by allowing me to reap more from my weight-training workouts, but it also improves all the activities in my day-to-day life. Most 250-pound guys would have an extremely difficult time on a hike, for example, because they're

carrying an extra 60 to 100 pounds of weight on their frames. But just last year, my wife and I took a long hike in Zion National Park, and I was able to reach the peak of our hike without gasping for air. We were able to talk, relax, and enjoy being in one of the most beautiful places in the world.

Even if you just want to be a better parent and family member, training multiple fitness skills is critical. It prevents you from becoming tired as you run up and down the sidelines coaching your kid's soccer game or when you move a new piece of furniture around the house until you find just the right place for it. It also improves your general health.

So, strive to become good at everything.

CARDIO MAKES YOU BIGGER AND STRONGER

Cardiovascular exercise is key, whether you're trying to be stronger or just live longer. Doing one or two long, slow runs, rides, rows, or swims each week can help you put on more muscle and increase your strength.

That's because a relaxed cardiovascular-based session helps your body recover between intense weight-lifting sessions. It works by increasing your blood flow and delivering more oxygen to your muscles. During a strength or power workout, you'll recover quicker between sets and won't become as fatigued, which means that you'll be able to get in more reps with heavier weights. After your workout, that boost in blood flow and oxygen delivery negates soreness and resets your central nervous system. You'll go into the rebuilding stage quicker, so that you can hit the gym hard again.

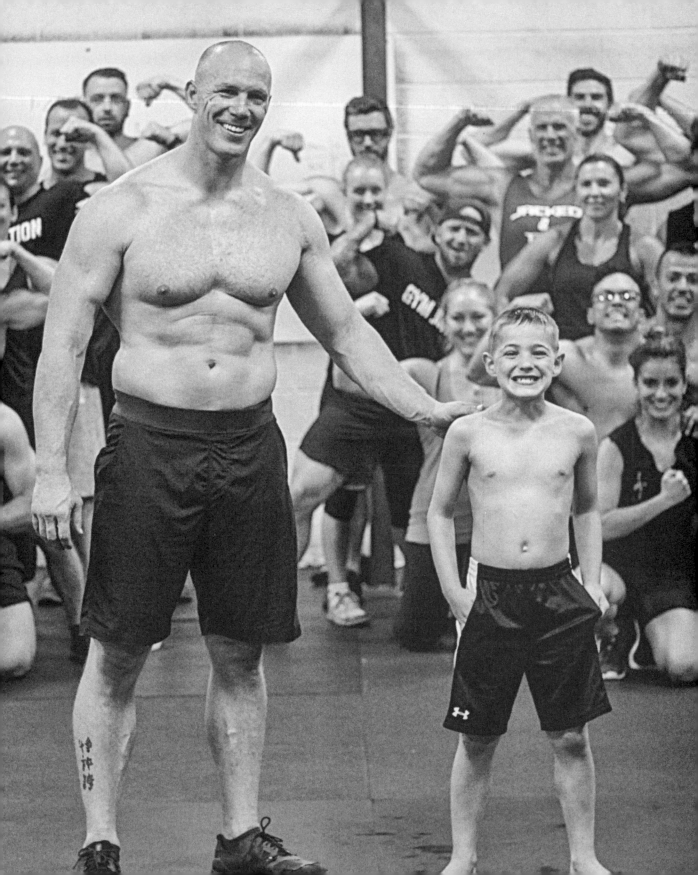

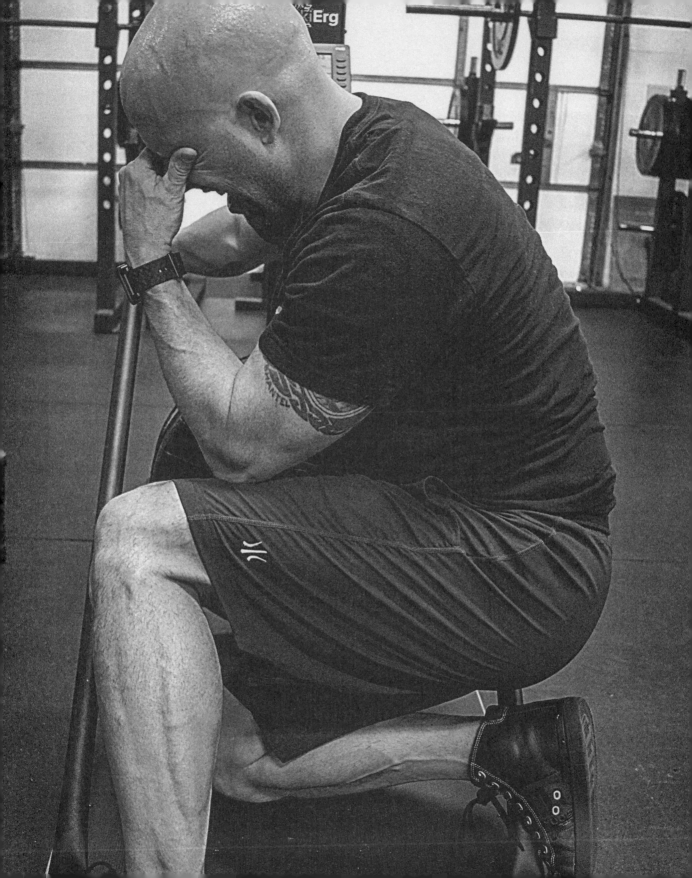

KILL YOUR GOVERNOR

If you've taken away anything by now, it's that hard work is what leads to real fitness and transformation, and it's your brain that needs to transform to allow you to work hard. That's not some theory I cooked up. Scientists have been studying the brain's impacts on exercise since the early 20th century.

Nobel Prize-winning scientist Archibald Hill, PhD, in 1924 first proposed the idea that your brain regulates exercise effort. He believed that your brain has a "governor" that prevents you from working so hard that you cause serious damage to your heart.

Hill's theory took more than 70 years to gain traction. It was overshadowed by the prevailing theory that the effort you can give is all about cellular supply and demand . . . that the only reason your muscles get tired is that they run out of fuel or build up too much lactic acid, causing you to slow down or stop altogether.

The problem: Scientists have never been able to prove that muscles receive too little oxygen or fuel during training. And another fact that hurts the theory is that even during the most intense exercise bouts, studies show, people rarely recruit more than 50 percent of their full muscle capacity. So what's the real issue?

Scientists call the answer to this problem the central governor theory. The theory states that your brain is responsible for determining how long, hard, and fast you push yourself as a mechanism to keep you safe from overexertion. During exercise, your brain is continually adjusting how much effort it allows you to give based on things like your past workouts, how long you're planning to exercise for, and your current physical state (for example, whether you're sick, didn't get much sleep, and so on).

A South African professor named Tim Noakes, MD, PhD, has been involved in numerous studies on the central governor theory. His conclusion from years and years of research on the topic: "Your brain sabotages your performance," says Dr. Noakes. "When you feel fatigued [during exercise], it's just an emotion. It has nothing to do with your physical state at all."

Other scientists agree with Dr. Noakes.

When Eduardo Fontes, PhD, a Brazil-based exercise scientist, had cyclists pedal to exhaustion while analyzing their brain activity on an fMRI machine, he showed that emotion plays a fundamental role in performance.[6] He says that he saw that these people's limbic lobes—the emotional centers of their brains light up as they increased exercise intensity and became more exhausted. The more active the limbic lobe became, the more emotion they tied to exertion, and the more they slowed. Your mental state, he explains, is behind much of the variation in your day-to-day performance.

Let's face it: Anyone who works out knows that performance can change drastically from one training session to the next. But physiologically, you probably haven't changed all that much; what can change from one session to the next is your mental state.

You've likely experienced the central governor yourself. Think back to high-school gym class, and your 2-mile run time test. You and your

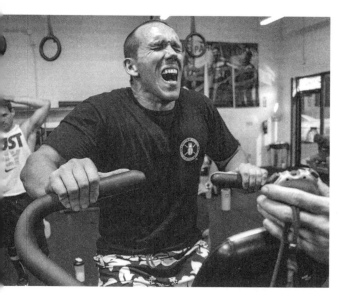

classmates lined up at your high-school's track. Your gym teacher yelled out "Eight laps as fast as you can! Go!" starting the stopwatch as you all took off.

The first lap you probably felt fine. This is easy. Not so bad. I can do this. Sometime into lap two, you noticed that your heart was beginning to beat at a fast pace and your breathing was becoming labored. You thought about the six-and-a-half laps you had left, and the finish line seemed like an impossibly long way away. You pressed on.

Then, somewhere between laps three and six, your central governor came in full bore. You noticed that your heart felt like it was going into cardiac arrest. Your legs? They felt like they were filled with battery acid. It was distressing, and it occurred to you that the multiple laps you had ahead of you may be insurmountable at this pace.

And so your brain sent you a loud-and-clear message: I need to slow down; I'm too tired to keep this pace. I can't keep running this fast. I'm going to get sick if I keep this up. I have to quit. You gave in and tapped the brakes, slowing down, completing your laps at that more comfortable pace.

Then something funny likely happened in the last stretches of your final lap. When you realized you had only one track-length ahead of you, you started to haul ass, running just as fast, if not faster, than you did off the starting line. You cruised to the finish line, and finished strong.

Wait a second. If you had done exactly what your teacher instructed—completed the eight laps as fast as possible—there's no way you would have been able to run any faster at the end. It's an impossibility: You should have maintained an equally fast pace throughout the run, and if you gave the test truly everything you had, you would likely have collapsed at the finish line.

What caused those wild swings in speed? Your brain. That screaming to "slow down!" and distressing fatigue all came from upstairs, and it sabotaged your performance.

Still, today, your central governor holds you back from working hard.

How do you kill your governor, so you can perform at your best and reach new heights in your fitness? The simplest, most-effective way is to understand the difference between exercise and training.

My friend Matt is a shining example of what happens when you begin to realize the difference between the two.

When I met Matt, he had a working knowledge of fitness. He'd deadlifted, rowed, and was experienced with kettlebells. He understood the difference between isometric and compound movements, and knew that HIIT (high-intensity interval training) wasn't a boxing move. Like most people, he made quick progress when he started working out. But then, like most people, he settled into a plateau. Even though he worked diligently with a few different trainers, he'd been stuck in the same fitness rut for a few years.

Bobby's Law:
No rest is taken except the rest that is earned.

He came to me for answers, and together we went over his typical workout routines. When I asked him about his goals and intention behind each workout, he replied that it was to get through it and try hard. Matt was only exercising.

I call it exercise when you go to the gym and do a bunch of stuff without having a tangible end point, beyond some abstract notion of fitness. You can't really work hard when you have no measurement of what hard work actually is.

So, I made Matt start training. Matt set a handful of fitness goals, and I wrote him a simple pro-gram. It consisted of just five workouts that he repeated on a weekly basis. Each workout had a very specific performance goal. The catch: Each time Matt did one of those workouts, he had to perform better than he did the last time.

Matt, for example, could deadlift 325 pounds, but declared that he wanted to lift 400. At the outset, pulling 400 pounds from the ground seemed like eons away. So instead, we made Matt's goal that day to deadlift 327.5 pounds. That seemed like no big deal to Matt. He could always lift 2.5 pounds more, right? And once he did, his very next session, his goal changed to 330, and so on. He was also rowing 2,000 meters in 7:20, but wanted to finish it below 7:00 minutes. Taking 20 seconds off his time was something that seemed far, far away and had always eluded him. And so, the first time he stepped into the gym after setting his goal, he attempted to row the distance in 7:19.5, and did.

He repeated that pattern of ever-so-slight progress each workout. A month in, Matt admitted something to me: He'd found a whole new level of intensity. What he'd been doing the past few years wasn't even close to pushing his limit.

Following that pattern, in a handful of months, Matt was able to row 2,000 meters in less than 7 minutes and was doing multiple deadlift repetitions at 365 pounds, which indicated he could easily deadlift more than 400 pounds for one rep.

What's more, Matt was also more athletic, could run faster and jump higher, and his body composition changed dramatically—the guy looked like a star athlete. At 40, he attained the highest level of fitness that he had had in his entire life. He's now such a fit person that I consider him a training partner rather than a trainee.

Follow Matt's lead: Break your primary goal into increments—and every time you repeat a workout, go just a little bit faster, lift slightly more, or do one more rep than you did the last workout. Don't push it—stick to small improvements.

Responsibility doesn't take days off.

When implemented consistently, this method has improved the performance of nearly every single person I've worked with. It's helped average guys hit my fitness standards, and it's helped pro athletes I work with run faster and jump higher.

The strategy works extremely well for three reasons. First, it forces you to start training, which is working out with a specific performance goal in mind (as opposed to simply going through "exercise" with an abstract ideal of where it'll take you).

Second, because large goals are daunting, this method gives each workout a micro goal. That makes each workout more purposeful and allows for continual improvement, which not only makes you fitter, it also builds your psychological resilience. Success breeds success.

Third, and perhaps most important, it kills your central governor and teaches you the feeling of hard work. I can tell you to work hard all day, but we all have a different definition of what hard work actually is. Cognitively, "work hard" is abstract. But something like "run 1 mile, 1 second faster than you did last time" is attainable. And run-

WHY I LOVE THE 2K ROW

Let me explain why I've mentioned the 2,000-meter row so often. Nearly everything I do is both a physical *and* psychological challenge. I want to put you in an uncomfortable position, so you reach the point where your mind tells you to give up. Then, I want you to dig deep and push on.

My favorite way to test—and build—your psychological will is to set a rowing machine for 2,000 meters, and have you go for time.

It works as a mind and body challenge because you can't cheat. The only way to gain an advantage is by pushing harder. The clock is unbiased and unforgiving. I encourage you to do this test once a month.

THE STANDARD: 7 MINUTES

Seven minutes tells me that you're not only in good shape, but that you're also willing to silence your mental demons, go all out, and keep getting better.

Of course, you should try to log the best time possible. I regularly see people finish in the low 6-minute range. (All other things being equal, taller, heavier people generally log faster times than shorter, lighter people.)

When you take this test, you'll probably think the first 500 meters is relatively easy. But halfway through, your mindset will change.

This is when your wheels begin to fall off, because you're left alone with your thoughts. I've watched numerous people go through this, and it quickly progresses from *I'm not going to make it* to *I'm going to die if I keep going.*

In fact, a good test of whether you're going hard enough is to ask yourself: Do I want to quit right now? If your answer is no, you aren't rowing hard enough.

I can tell you this: If you fight to the end, you'll become something more. The people who succeed are always better for it, and it usually unlocks the door to success in many other areas of their training.

THE HARDEST WORKOUT I'VE EVER DONE

You never forget your first SMMF, or single movement mind f*ck. It's exactly what it sounds like—one exercise repeated over and over again until you finish, quit, or go batshit crazy. It puts you in a state of serious physical and psychological stress. But if you finish strong, it'll forever change the way you work out.

My first SMMF was on New Year's Day of 2009. I was visiting family in Canada. All of the gyms were closed, and my mom had no fitness equipment in the house. So I went to the laundry room, which was the only unoccupied room in her house and just big enough to fit the washer, the dryer, and me.

Then I did 2,009 lunges. It was the definition of terrible. My legs burned. My body shook. My mind went hazy. It felt like torture, and there were multiple moments that I wanted to throw in the towel. I kept going, though, until I finished the last rep 2 hours later.

I'm glad I finished. After that SMMF, other tough workouts didn't seem all that bad. I gained a never-say-die mantra, pushing harder, setting loftier goals, and reaching new heights in my fitness.

Want to try a SMMF? A few of my favorites: Do 1,000 lunges facing a wall (much worse than outside or in front of the TV) or carry two 32-kilo or 70-pound dumbbells for 1 mile.

ning just 1 second faster? Not that hard. Over time, you understand what hard work feels like and find your true limits, and the improvements add up.

I've had people I train apply this strategy to more than just their workouts. They've used it to sleep more (go to bed 1 minute earlier) and improve their nutrition (eat just one less piece of candy a day). It's also incredibly effective for your recovery practices, which you'll learn about in the next section. If foam rolling for 10 minutes a night—like I suggest—sounds like too much, start with just 30 seconds.

Doing just a little better than you did last time is a no-stress proposition that allows you to override your central governor. Try it. Improve. Thank me later.

Bobby's Law:
Our biggest fears carry with them the greatest opportunity for personal growth.

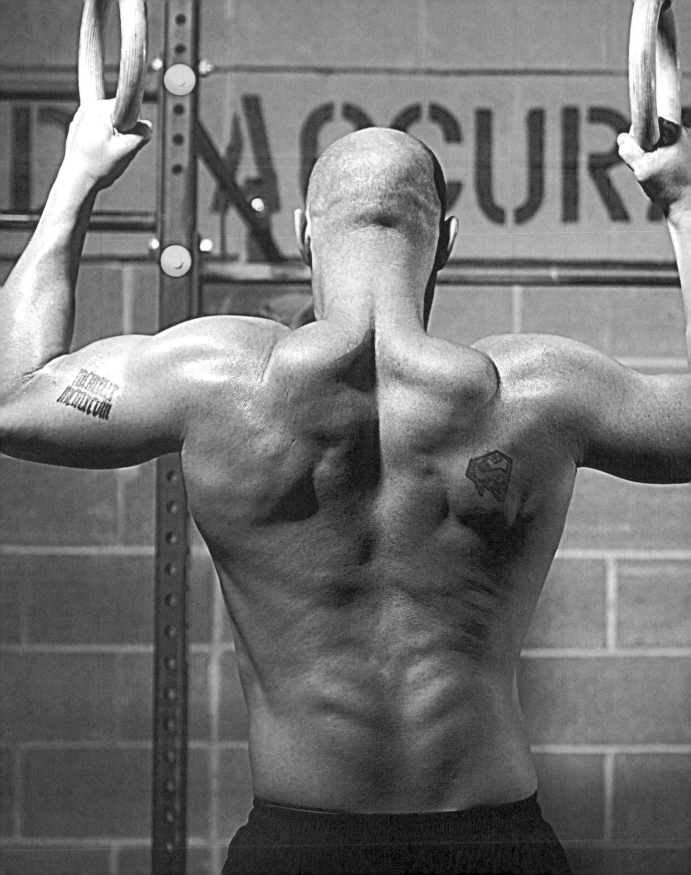

SUPPORT

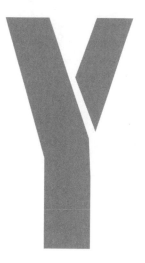

You may have heard people talk about a condition called overtraining. The theory is that if you train too hard, too often, and don't recover fully from each session, your body begins to break down. Symptoms include insomnia, chronic pain, depression, irritability, abnormal heart rate, illness, and more.

Today, the condition is hilariously rampant—anyone who regularly goes to the gym and has ever had a headache, sad thought, or sore muscles has probably been told they might be overtraining. The fix, people are told, is to work out less, or to not train as intensely.

The reality: Most people don't train with enough intensity to even come close to being overtrained. If you've ever reduced the volume or the intensity of your workouts because you think you're overtraining, you've only sabotaged yourself. Here's why: There is no such thing as overtraining. There is only underrecovery.

Anyone who's ever suffered from overtraining-like symptoms (keep in mind this usually only happens to people who train 15 or more hours a week) has come down with the conditions because he or she neglected some facet of his or her recovery from their training: Their nutrition was off, they weren't sleeping enough, they had too much stress in their lives, or they weren't taking care of their bodies.

When someone tells me that they think they're overtraining, I tell them about Hack's Pack. The CrossFit Games are a war of attrition. In the Games, 40 individual men and women and teams perform approximately 13 brutal workouts over the course of 5 days to determine who is the fittest man, woman, and team of people on Earth.

In a typical day at the CrossFit Games, the athletes might do a workout where they wear a 20-pound weight vest as they run a mile, do 100 pullups, 200 pushups, and 300 squats, and then run another mile (a workout named Murph). After that, they might do a barbell complex of deadlifts, power cleans, and jerks with hundreds of pounds on the bar. Then they might do a couple of sprint workouts or a 75-minute row. It's an incredibly demanding competition.

In 2012 and 2013, I trained Hack's Pack, a six-person squad from Ute CrossFit that competed in the team competition of the games. They trained in the gym for 15 to 20 hours a week, and each hour was spent at full tilt. Their training program included everything you see in the CrossFit Games: running, jumping, sprinting, heavy lifting, rowing, gymnastics, Olympic lifts, and more. Yet somehow, they never became overtrained. Why?

I hammered home to them this point: Recovery is half of the battle. If you neglect recovery, it'll take you exceedingly more time and effort to reach your goal.

Training hard places stress on your system and tears up your muscles. It's actually when you're outside of the gym when your body works to recover from this stress and damage, repair your muscles, and improve its fitness. The faster you can recover, the quicker you can train hard again and progress.

That's why I made sure that Hack's Pack was extremely diligent with their nutrition and recovery and used the everyday strategies you're about to learn about in this section.

The more they paid attention to their nutrition, and the harder they worked with their recovery practices, the better they became. When it came time to go to the CrossFit Games, that attention paid off.

After the first couple workouts of 2012's competition, Hack's Pack found themselves in the middle of the running. But after those two workouts, things changed: Hack's Pack was fresh and fully recovered and able to perform normally, while every other team was tired and began to perform at a deficit. Hack's Pack took first place in four of the remaining nine workouts, and they didn't finish below seventh place in the five others. They won the team competition that year.

The same thing happened the next year. In fact, in 2013, they were so far ahead in points by the last workout that they didn't even have to participate.

After each win, they told me that their attention to properly refueling and recovering was the difference maker. It not only allowed them to improve more before the games but, more importantly, it also allowed them to recover faster between workouts so that they could go harder in each successive event.

If you're working hard in the gym and not actively helping your body refuel and repair, you're

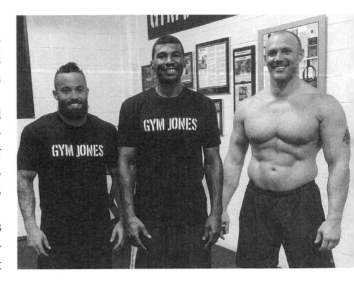

sabotaging your results. I used these nutrition and recovery practices with Hack's Pack, but I also use them with every single person who comes through the gym, from people trying to shed fat to those competing in an endurance event. They're the key to taking your fitness to the next level.

Think of it this way: There are 168 hours in a week. Even if you train 10 hours a week, you still have 158 hours a week to screw it all up by eating poorly, neglecting your sleep, making poor lifestyle decisions, and not taking care of your body. What you do outside of the gym is often the determining factor of whether you reach a fitness goal or not.

You may be surprised to find that my nutrition rules are shockingly straightforward, and are centered on personal responsibility. I'm not going to tell you exactly what to eat, I'm going to give you the information you need to find the right diet for you.

You'll learn five strategies that rejuvenate your body between workouts. These methods not only allow you to reach your goals faster but they also increase your quality of life exponentially by reducing your stress, nixing any nagging pains you have, and boosting your energy across the board.

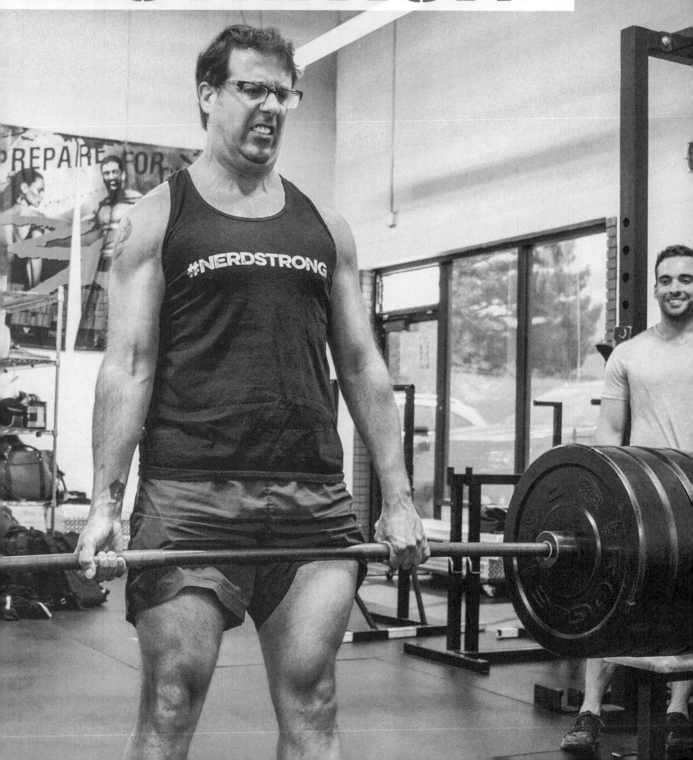

9

EAT TO SUPPORT YOUR GOAL

Most nights, I eat dinner at one of Salt Lake City's finest burger joints. My go-to meal is a double-patty burger and fries.

If I'm eating dinner at home, it's a 16-ounce steak topped with a pat of butter, with a beer and Doritos on the side. Sometimes, if I need a snack in a pinch, I'll stop at an In-N-Out burger for their grilled four-by-four, which, as the name implies, is a burger with four patties and four slices of cheese on it.

I like to post photos of these meals to Instagram. When I do, commenters inevitably have two reactions. The first reaction is amazement and a bit of good-natured jealousy that I'm able to eat those kinds of foods yet stay lean and hit my fitness goals. The second reaction isn't so nice. People attack my food choices, writing things like "your insides are rotting," "you eat like an idiot," or "you are going to get fat."

Here's what those negative people need to understand about my diet: My goal is to be the "Big Guy." I've spent nearly 20 years trying to get as big

as possible while staying lean. I'm 6 feet 3 inches, weigh 255 pounds, and have 9 percent body fat. I train hard—very hard—twice a day, 6 days a week, and I'm always trying to put on more muscle.

Just to maintain my weight and perform well in the gym, I need to eat 5,000 to 6,000 calories a day. But because I'm trying to add weight, I typically eat around 8,000.

Do you know how hard it is to take in 8,000 calories each day in only healthy foods? Even if I were to eat 10 pounds of chicken breast and 10 pounds of broccoli, I'd still be approximately 2,000 calories short of my goal.

I also don't think it would be physically possible to eat that much chicken and broccoli. I'd run out of room in my stomach, and it would take me all day to eat that food.

Indeed, healthy foods have a lot of volume for just a handful calories. That's great if you're trying to lose weight. The foods allow you to eat a lot, feel full, and yet stay within your daily calorie goals. But if you need a significant amount of calories,

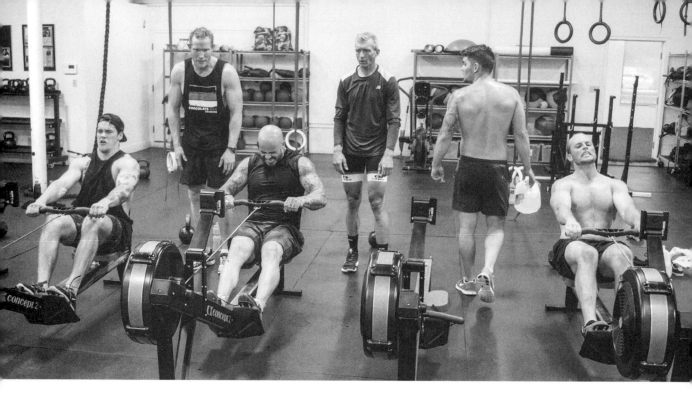

eating 100 percent healthy foods alone usually just doesn't cut it.

My calorie-packed nightly burger and fries, or steak, butter, and Doritos is the easiest way I can hit my caloric needs. A bag of Doritos, for example, has 1,400 calories, and it's incredibly easy to finish in a single sitting.

I'm not saying that what I'm doing is healthy. It's not. There is a big difference between eating to be generally healthy and eating to perform better or look a certain way. Fitness and aesthetic goals aren't always conducive to improving your general health.

Take, for example, my goal of being as big and muscle-bound as possible. My heart has to work harder to deliver more blood to my muscle, the amount of food I eat makes my other organs work harder, and my extra weight puts more stress on my joints.

I understand that and accept that as part of the cost of being the Big Guy.

Another thing that's critical to know about my diet: It doesn't consist *entirely* of burgers and fries, steaks and pats of butter, and bags of Doritos. What I don't post on Instagram is all the healthy food I eat, like fruits, nuts, lean meats, protein shakes, and vegetables. But the truth is that those foods are all an even bigger part of my diet because they deliver the vitamins, minerals, and nutrients I need to train hard, recover, and grow bigger. I don't post Instagram photos of those foods, because, honestly, where's the fun in posting pictures of spinach, kale, carrots, and almonds? There are plenty of instafamous yogis who've cornered the market on those types of posts.

Now, if your own goal is to become bigger, and you think I just gave you free license to eat burgers and Doritos every night so long as you also throw in some health foods, think again. Unless you have a body similar to mine and train as often and hard as I do, you'd just put on a lot of fat. The fact is that 99 percent of people just can't eat like I do.

Your diet has to be individualized to your own body and lifestyle, and it has to align with your goal. Everyone has a different body type, genetics, and lifestyle when it comes to work, exercise, sleep habits, and eating preferences. Different fitness goals require different diets—is your goal to perform well in a sport, or to just be generally healthier? Is your goal to gain, lose, or maintain your weight?

A 250-pound NFL linebacker has different needs compared to a 150-pound accountant who sits all day. An NFL linebacker needs to eat to be big, strong, and incredibly fast and powerful. Ideally, the accountant eats in a way that promotes his health and doesn't cause him to gain fat.

What's more, even if you take two people who, on paper, look exactly the same, things can be different. Resting metabolic rate—which is the number of calories you burn each day just to exist, breathe, think, and live—can vary up to 15 percent among people. That means one 210-pound guy might burn 300 more daily calories than another 210-pound guy without moving a single muscle.

Most people overcomplicate their diets, or look for magic foods and diets that promise to give them results in just a couple of weeks. But eating the right amount of food so that you'll see the results you want is simple, it just takes a little patience. Move too fast, and you'll only burn out, feel like crap, or put on fat.

First, determine about how much you should be eating: Estimate your calorie needs based on your weight, age, and activity levels. Multiple Web sites allow you to calculate this online, or you can see the "Calculate Your Calories" box below for a simple way to figure out a rough estimate. The numbers you calculate are general guidelines—you might actually need more or less food—but they're a good place to start. (You'll learn what specific foods you should eat later in this section.)

Try to eat the calorie goal provided for 2 to 4 weeks. To do this accurately, you'll have to track how many calories you eat each day. A calorie-counting app can be an easy way to do this. Try to be as precise as possible as you track your food. You could even use a food scale, if you wanted. Why? You'll determine your true needs and also learn a lot about your eating patterns and the

CALCULATE YOUR CALORIES

When I need to quickly estimate how many calories someone should eat in a day, I use these formulas.

If you are sedentary (little to no exercise):
Multiply your body weight in pounds by 10 to 13
If you exercise a moderate amount (3 to 5 times a week for an hour each session):
Multiply your body weight in pounds by 13 to 16
If you exercise a high amount (5 to 10 times a week for an hour or more each session):
Multiply your body weight in pounds by 16 to 20

So, for example, if you're a 180-pound guy who exercises for 1 hour, 4 times a week, you'd eat 2,340 to 2,880 calories each day.

These are simply rough targets and don't take into account your body fat percentage or your individualized specific goals. That's why you see a wide range in calories from the lowest recommendation to the highest.

true calorie cost of your favorite foods.

During that 2 to 4 weeks, keep track of what happens to your body. Did you gain weight? Did you lose weight? Did your fitness increase? Did nothing happen?

If, after your 2- to 4-week trial, your weight or performance didn't head in the direction that you wanted it to, add or subtract calories from your original calorie figure.

Don't do anything too extreme. Remember, intensity is the inverse of duration. If your goal is to lose weight, take 100 to 300 calories away from your calorie number. For a lot of people, this can simply be switching from a daily soda to a glass of unsweetened tea, or eating half of your normal dessert.

If your goal is to gain weight or to perform better, add in 100 to 300 calories. My suggestion: Drink a protein shake every day. A great option is "My Favorite Quick Muscle Shake" on page 84. It has a nice balance of protein, carbs, and fat, and it's easy to make in a pinch.

In another 2 to 4 weeks, reassess. If you've moved toward your goal, stay at that number of calories, and reassess every 2 to 4 weeks. Follow this pattern until you hit your goal, then stay at that level of calories. Continue to make assessments every 4 weeks or so.

Two things you should keep in mind: First, if you increase your activity level, you'll likely need to change how much you eat. For example, if you find that 2,700 calories suits you each day when you're training for 5 hours a week, you're probably going to have to bump that number up if you decide to tackle

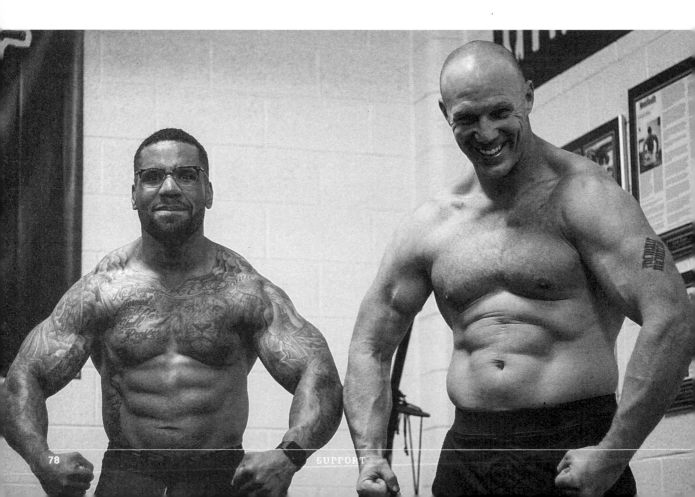

SUPPORT

6 WAYS TO EAT TO LOSE OR GAIN WEIGHT

Now that you know, generally, how to find your caloric needs, here are three tips that I give for each type of client to help them hit their calorie goals.

TO LOSE FAT

1. Don't drink your calories; drinks don't fill you up but they count toward your (low) calorie goal.
2. Don't eat any food within 3 hours of going to bed. You're most likely to snack mindlessly on junk foods after dinner, when you're relaxing.
3. Don't eat more than 500 calories in any single sitting. This makes each meal equally filling, so you won't ever become too hungry and binge.

TO GAIN MUSCLE

1. Drink your calories. Don't go overboard by pounding soda, but drinking a liquid like a protein shake or glass of milk each day adds valuable protein and calories without filling you up.
2. Eat a bedtime snack. This is an easy way to take in more calories.
3. Snack throughout the day. Chances are that you won't be able to meet your caloric needs in just three meals.

a marathon and begin to log 10 hours of weekly exercise. The same rule applies in reverse: Cut down your training, cut down your calories.

Second, keep track of how you look in the mirror. If your goal is simply to look better naked, trading fat for muscle is perfectly aligned with your goal, but your scale weight may not change. If you want to be more precise, you can have your body composition measured. Many gyms will do this for you for free, or, for a more exact number, you can go to a health facility that offers a DXA scan, an x-ray analysis that delivers the most accurate calculation of your body-fat percentage.

The above method takes a little longer than most crash diets advertise—it may take you a few months to figure out the perfect calorie number for you, and perhaps only then will you start to see significant results. But it's the right way. It's sustainable, and it lessens your chances of putting on fat because you eat too much, or feeling like crap because you eat too little, and, in turn, giving up along the way.

10

EAT REAL FOOD

Have you ever found yourself hungry, at a gas station, looking for something healthy to snack on? It's a nightmare. The aisles are filled with hundreds of food options, and every single one is processed, packaged, and chock-full of chemicals.

Look at an ingredients label, and you'll find words like "polysorbate 60," "diglycerides," and "calcium sulfate." The first is an emulsifier mostly used in cosmetics, the second a synthetic fat used often in packaged baked goods, and the third a desiccant mainly used in plaster.

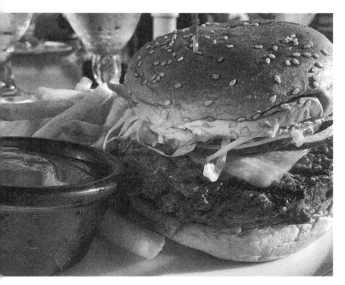

Chemical additives in food are all FDA approved, which means the Food and Drug Administration says that they won't do you any harm. But some chemicals are controversial, and the fact of the matter is that we don't know the long-term effects caused by consuming them. I'm not a scientist nor do I claim to be an expert on the subject, but when it comes to my body, I'd rather be safe than sorry. Even if I could be assured that eating silicone or calcium sulfate isn't bad for me, I also know that they aren't giving me much of a nutritional benefit or fitness boost.

So, I favor eating real food. I have a handful of rules I use to determine if a food is real: If it was available to eat 150 years ago, it's real. If you can kill it or pluck it from the ground, then it's real. If I can visualize the ingredients, it's real. (I know, for example, what a tomato or grapefruit looks like, but have no clue what a soy lecithin looks like.)

You don't have to be militant about this. If you occasionally eat something that includes a chemical or comes in a package, that's okay. Some packaged foods can help you reach your goal. Canned and bagged vegetables, beans, and fish are great for you. The key is that none of those have anything extra added to the can or bag except for

IS IT WORTH IT TO EAT ORGANIC?

I know people who put premium fuel in their European luxury sedan, but won't spend a few extra cents on higher-quality fuel for the most important vehicle they own: their bodies. People complain that organic and higher-quality food is too expensive, but there are a handful of simple methods you can use to save money.

ORDER MEAT ONLINE

There are various Web sites that deliver grass-fed, organic meat to your door for a fraction of the price you'd pay for the same product at the grocery store.

BUY IN BULK AND FREEZE

Wait for sales and stock up on an item, or purchase a membership to a bulk-discount store like Costco. You'll pay more up front but will save money in the long run.

GO LOCAL

Local farmers often use far less pesticides on their crops compared with factory farms. What's more, you'll also pay less, and your produce will taste better.

THE CLEAN 15

Avocados, sweet corn, pineapples, cabbage, frozen sweet peas, onions, asparagus, mangoes, papayas, kiwi fruits, eggplant, honeydew melons, grapefruit, cantaloupe, and cauliflower

THE DIRTY DOZEN

Strawberries, apples, nectarines, peaches, celery, grapes, cherries, spinach, tomatoes, sweet bell peppers, cherry tomatoes, and cucumbers

BUY THE "CLEAN 15" CONVENTIONAL, AND THE "DIRTY DOZEN" ORGANIC

Each year, the Environmental Working Group provides a list of the cleanest and dirtiest fruits and vegetables. The Clean 15 generally have the fewest pesticides, while the Dirty Dozen have the most. That means that the difference between a Clean 15 vegetable that's organic versus conventional isn't that big, while the difference between a Clean 15 versus organic Dirty Dozen vegetable is significant.

maybe some water and salt. And I think we can all agree that protein powder comes in a package and wasn't around 150 years ago. But most people have a hard time reaching their daily protein goal, which holds back their results. Drinking a protein shake every day is a convenient way to reach your protein goal.

Foods like Doritos and drive-thru burgers are obviously not "real food," but even they can have a place in your diet—within moderation. (You'll soon learn how to fit those foods into your diet with "Follow the Maximus 90-Percent Rule" on page 92.)

My Doritos, for example, have nothing remotely "real" about them. It's a fried tortilla blasted with neon nacho cheese-flavored powder. But, again, I simply can't consume all my calories from healthy, real foods.

Remember, I'm getting most of my calories from real food (sure, steak and butter were around 150 years ago, as were the beef, bread, and cheese that make up my homemade burgers).

You may find this method hard at first, but once you start to follow it, and real foods start to fill your kitchen, you'll find it's actually not that difficult. Most important is that you'll likely feel better, more fully, and will wish you'd cut out chemical-laden, processed foods earlier.

11

EAT IN BALANCE

There are hundreds of fad diets. Most of them ask you to avoid something: carbs, fats, meats, animal products, gluten, nightshades, foods a caveman wouldn't eat. This list goes on.

These diets rarely last. Remember in the 1990s when fat was vilified and "low-fat" was king? Back then, eating fat was blamed for all kinds of health issues, ranging from heart disease to obesity. People, in turn, cut fat and began eating more carbohydrates.

Then, sometime in the early 2000s, the thinking did a 180-degree turn. Carbohydrates are now the bad guy, responsible for diabetes, obesity, and every other problem you can think of.

Diets that ask you to cut out entire food groups or give you a list of "good" and "bad" foods tend to fail most people because they're not sustainable. For one, I've found that there's some strange psychology behind saying you'll never eat anything that actually makes that food more appealing to you. For another, these diets make it hard to eat socially. What do you do if you're on the Paleo diet, and your daughter wants to have her birthday at a pizza place? You either don't eat or you find some way to piece together menu items into a Paleo-approved meal.

Eating a balanced diet filled with real foods makes eating healthier much easier, and therefore much more sustainable. That approach also ensures that you're consuming enough of the nutrients you need to reach your goal, whether that's to lose weight, build muscle, or perform better. Indeed, there's a strong argument—no matter your goal—for making sure that you eat the three basic macronutrients: protein, fats, and carbohydrates.

PROTEIN

Protein is your body's main building block. Your body needs protein to grow, repair your tissues, produce hormones, boost your immune system, and—most important when it comes to fitness goals—to build and maintain your muscle mass.

For most people who exercise, eating about 1 gram of protein per pound of body weight is ideal. So, let's say you weigh 180 pounds. If you want to lose weight or maintain your current weight, you'd eat about 180 grams each day.

There's a good reason why you should eat a lot

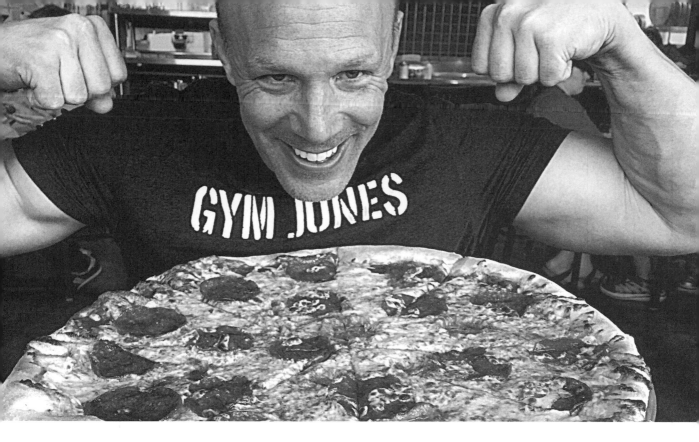

of protein when you're trying to lose weight: It can help you cut fat and build muscle, according to a study in the *American Journal of Clinical Nutrition.*[1]

The scientists took 40 overweight guys and had them each do an intense, 6-day-a-week training routine that consisted of total-body lifting sessions, high-intensity circuits, and explosive body-weight exercises. The participants all ate 40 percent fewer calories than they needed to maintain their current weights (that's not much food). The primary factor that scientists manipulated was protein. Half the participants ate about 15 percent of their calories from protein, while the other half took in 35 percent from protein. The latter number was equivalent to the participants eating about 1 gram of protein per pound of their body weights.

When the 4-week study was up, both groups had lost about 11 pounds. But where that weight came from is the key to the study. The low-protein group lost that weight from a mix of body fat and muscle. The high-protein group, on the other hand, actually gained 3 pounds of muscle, meaning that nearly all of the 11 pounds they lost was from fat. When you lose fat and gain muscle, two things happen: Your body composition improves, so you look better, and your fitness improves.

If you want to bulk up, go ahead and eat more protein—a good rule of thumb for adding muscle is to eat your goal weight in grams. For example, if you're 180 pounds and you'd like to go up to 200 pounds, then aim to eat about 200 grams of protein.

No matter your goal, eat at least 30 grams per

MY FAVORITE QUICK MUSCLE SHAKE

If I'm ever pressed for time and need to quickly slam some quality nutrition, I make this shake. It takes about 30 seconds to shake up in a blender bottle, and it delivers a great mix of nutrients.

1 cup 100% orange juice
1 tablespoon high-quality fish oil
1 scoop vanilla whey protein

Nutrition: 350 calories, 29 grams carbs, 15 grams fat, 24 grams protein

meal. That number maxes out your body's ability to repair muscle. It also makes it easier to nail your overall protein goal if you're taking in a higher number each meal.

In general, try to consume your protein from a variety of real sources like meats, yogurt, and nuts. But, as mentioned, whey powder may not have been around 150 years ago, but it's an incredibly helpful resource that allows you to hit your daily protein goal. Don't be afraid to use it.

FATS

In 1998, when I wrestled in college, my coach wanted me to compete in the 285-pound weight class. I weighed about 215 at the time.

I wanted that 70-pound increase to be from as much muscle as possible. So, I altered my training and I adopted a standard, low-fat bodybuilder diet. This was during the apex of the low-fat craze, and everything I read told me that eating fat would make me fat. Many items in the grocery store came in a normal version and a low-fat or fat-free version. So my grocery list was filled with the latter options.

About a month in, I just wasn't adding the muscle I wanted to. What's more, I also felt run down and tired, and my gym performance was suffering. I struggled to figure out my problem, until one day it occurred to me that I started to feel bad around the time that I cut out fat. So, I took a chance and added fat back into my diet, keeping my overall calories high.

Nearly immediately, I started to feel and perform better, and add the muscle that I needed to compete.

Besides tasting great, fats are necessary for you to survive. They help you grow, give you energy, and maintain healthy cell, brain, lung, hormone levels, and immune function, plus they allow you to absorb more nutrients from the foods you eat, like vegetables.

There's no definitive rule on how much fat you should eat, but a rule of thumb I use is to aim to take in half of your body weight in grams of fat. So, our 180-pound guy should eat about 90 grams per day, from mostly unprocessed sources.

Generally, unsaturated fats are the healthiest. They come from nuts, seeds, olive oils, fish, and avocados. Scientists say that these types of fats may help you avoid heart disease, lower your cholesterol levels, and more.

Next in line are saturated fats—fats that mostly occur naturally in animal products like meats, eggs, cheeses, yogurt, and other dairy products. Years ago, flawed research created a myth that saturated fats led to heart disease—which is why, for a while, we all thought that egg yolks and steak would clog our arteries. But a recent study review and a massive scientific consensus meeting at the University of Copenhagen determined that saturated fat doesn't need to be avoided because there's no clear link to saturated fats and heart disease.[2]

In fact, many studies have found that eating saturated fat can improve your liver function, enhance your immune system, and—most important when you train hard—boost your testosterone levels, helping you recover from workouts and repair and build muscle faster.

Always avoid trans fats, which are chemically created fats. In fact, the Institute of Medicine says that trans fats have no health benefits, aren't safe at any level, and should be avoided. That's because—among many things—they create inflammation, which can lead to heart disease, diabetes, stroke, and other health problems. Research from the Harvard T. H. Chang School of Public Health suggests that for every 2 percent of your calories that come from trans fats—that's 4 grams if you eat 2,000 calories a day—your risk of heart disease rises by 23 percent.[3]

You'll find trans fats primarily in fried fast foods, margarine, and a lot of packaged goods like cookies, cakes, pies, and microwave popcorn.

CARBOHYDRATES

Low carb is the new low fat. Sometime in the late 1990s or early 2000s, the low-carb diet took off. Some experts estimate that, at the diet's peak, 18 percent of the population was eating some form of the low-carbohydrate diet.

I've also tried eating low carb. I lost weight, and it may help you lose weight, too. But, for me, I'm not entirely sure if I lost weight due to cutting carbs or simply by cutting out the calories that came from carbs.

You may have heard that carbs make you put on weight. Some people may be sensitive to carbs, but multiple studies show that carbs don't have some magic ability to make you fat. A study published in the *American Journal of Clinical Nutrition* found that there wasn't any real difference in terms of weight loss and muscle-to-fat ratios of people who followed a low-carb diet versus those who followed a high-carb diet.[4] Another study found that there's no difference in metabolism between people who eat lower- and higher-carb diets.[5]

Overeating carbs, not the carbs themselves, primarily makes you fat. That can happen if you overeat fat or protein, too. But what makes carbs unique is that they're far easier to overeat compared to the other two macronutrients.

For example, there are 1,000 calories in 50 Starburst candies, nearly all of which are from carbs. There are also 1,000 calories in about 2 pounds of boneless skinless chicken breast, which is basically pure protein. I think we can agree that sitting down and eating 50 Starburst candies in a row would not only be quick and easy, it would also be enjoyable. Eating 2 pounds of boneless skinless chicken breast in one sitting, on the other hand, would be one of the blandest, most arduous experiences of your life. You probably wouldn't want to eat chicken for the next month by the time you finished.

Carbohydrates also tend to be hidden in many of the junk foods we eat, in the form of sugar. For example, peanut butter and fruit-flavored yogurt have sugar added to them.

So, once you start paying attention to your carb intake, it only make sense that your calories might drop, and that you'll lose weight. But if your goal is to perform better, or maintain or gain weight, being too carb conscious can be problematic. I've found that some people who train hard and avoid carbs actually eat too few calories, in general, and don't have enough fuel. Add carbs back in, and these people instantly perform better.

Carbohydrates and protein each have 4 calories per gram, while a gram of fat has 9 calories. Follow the advice to eat about 1 gram of protein and 0.5 gram of fat per pound of your body weight, and simply make the rest of your calories carbs. So, for example, let's say you're that 180-pound guy, and you've determined that you need to eat about 2,500 calories every day to maintain your weight and perform at your peak. You'd eat:

Protein: 180 grams, which is a total of 720 calories

Fat: 90 grams, which is a total of 810 calories

So you're up to 1,530 calories. Do the math (2,500 minus 1,530) and you have about 970 calories left. That means that you should eat about 240 grams of carbs each day (that number is 970 divided by 4, the number of calories in 1 gram of carbohydrates).

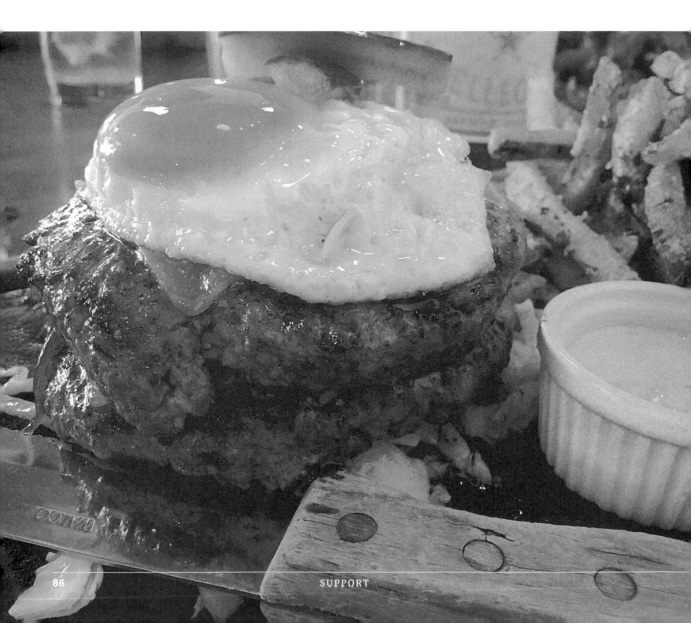

PUTTING IT ALL TOGETHER

To help you see what your diet plan looks like spread across an average day, here's a sample eating plan for a 180-pound person who requires 2,500 calories a day.

BREAKFAST	CALORIES	CARBS	FAT	PROTEIN
Oatmeal, ½ cup, cooked	150	27	3	6
Eggs, jumbo, 3 (65 g)	288	2	20	25
Walnuts, 0.5 oz	94	2	9	2
Blueberries, 1 cup	85	21	1	1
TOTAL	**617**	**52**	**33**	**34**
LUNCH				
Side salad	25	5	0	1
Ancient grain spelt bread, 2 slices	220	38	5	8
Roasted turkey breast, 4 oz	120	0	2	26
Banana, 1	105	27	0	1
Swiss cheese, 1 slice (18 g)	70	0	5	5
TOTAL	**540**	**70**	**12**	**41**
DINNER				
Russet potato, 1	110	26	0	3
Sour cream, 2 Tbsp (30 g)	60	2	5	1
Broccoli, steamed, 1 cup	47	9	1	4
Steak, skirt, 8 oz	477	0	24	61
TOTAL	**694**	**37**	**30**	**69**
SNACKS				
Almond butter, 1 packet (1.15 oz, 32 g) or 2 Tbsp	200	6	18	6
Apple, McIntosh, 1 medium	80	22	0	0
100% whey protein, 1.5 scoops	180	5	2	36
Tangerines, 5 small	200	50	0	3
TOTAL	**660**	**83**	**20**	**45**
TOTALS	**2,511**	**242**	**95**	**189**

You don't have to eat exactly these foods, of course. I just want to give you a sense of what your meals may look like under my general recommendations. If you find that you look, feel, and perform best on, say, a Paleo diet, by all means, go ahead and eat Paleo. The best diet is always the one that you'll stick to and that fits into your lifestyle.

12

EAT OFTEN

Calories are king. You can eat any way you want to, on any diet you choose. As long as you eat the right amount of calories from a good mix of healthy foods, and you train hard, you'll nail your goal. This strategy has worked for literally every single person that I've worked with.

You could eat two massive meals a day that fulfill all of your calorie and macronutrient needs and reach your goal. Conversely, you could eat all of your calories and macros across 20 meals and also reach your goal.

But I tell most people to eat five or six smaller meals a day. Here's why: It becomes difficult to keep meals small enough if you eat seven or more daily. And eating just two meals a day makes it hard to eat enough calories every day, and, more important, resist temptations that pop up when you're hungry.

Intense hunger derails your willpower. When you're starving, you're more likely to stop for fast food on the way home from work, eat the brownies your colleague baked for the office, or shove kettle-cooked barbecue chips into your face as you wait for your healthy dinner to cook.

The best way to avoid that intense hunger is to eat every 3 to 4 hours throughout the day. By doing this, you're basically just limiting the possibility that you'll eat unplanned (typically unhealthy) foods. The math works out to five or six meals a day.

WHY PEOPLE CALL ME "MAXIMUS"

When I was in college, I needed to eat a ton of calories so I could gain weight to wrestle in the heavyweight division. But, as a college student, I didn't have much money for a big grocery bill.

To supplement my diet, I started eating a jar of peanut butter a day. For just a few bucks, it gave me 2,670 calories. I'd walk around campus all day eating from the jar, so the captain of our wrestling team nicknamed me "PB." Soon, everyone was calling me that.

But, after the peanut butter trick started working and I put on a lot of muscle, people began calling me "PB Maximus." As the "Big Guy," I started winning most of my matches, and the wrestling team dropped "PB" and just started calling me "Maximus." The name stuck for good.

It doesn't really matter how you spread the calories out across those meals. Let's say you eat 2,500 calories a day. You could split that into five meals of 500 calories. Or, you could eat a 500-calorie breakfast, a 500-calorie lunch, a couple of 200-calorie snacks, and a 1,100-calorie dinner. You'd make equivalent progress using either approach—simply experiment and see what works best for you.

One thing to note: This method won't boost your metabolism any more than would eating three square meals a day. You may have heard that eating five or six small meals a day will "stoke your metabolic fire," or that "skipping meals causes you to store fat."

Many studies have shown that that old idea isn't true. For example, a *British Journal of Nutrition* review looked at all the studies on the topic and concluded that increasing the frequency of your meals has zero effect on your metabolism.[6]

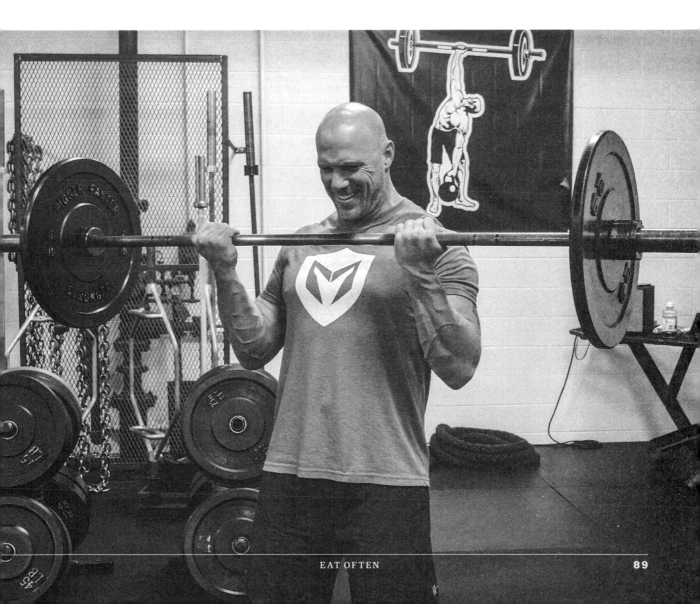

13

ENJOY YOURSELF

I've worked with and been friends with Tommy Hackenbruck for years. He was the middle linebacker for the 2004 University of Utah Utes squad that was arguably the best college football team in the country that year. They went undefeated and won the Fiesta Bowl. Urban Meyer was that team's coach, and Alex Smith was its quarterback.

After graduating from the University of Utah, Tommy became interested in CrossFit. He opened a few CrossFit boxes in Salt Lake City, called Ute CrossFit, and has been competing in the games ever since.

Tommy is one of the best athletes I've ever met. He's one of those guys that's really good at any sport or physical task you give him. He can deadlift 535 pounds, back squat 525 pounds, do 50 pullups in a row, and run 400 meters in less than a minute.

Tommy is 6 feet 1 inch tall and 205 pounds. That's big for a competitive CrossFit athlete. Rich Froning, who won the CrossFit Games four times in a row, for example, is 5 feet 9 inches and about 195 pounds.

As I was training Tommy for the 2011 CrossFit Games, I thought that making him lighter would help him improve at the gymnastics moves in Cross-Fit competitions, such as pullups and muscle-ups. Generally, weighing less makes you better at body-weight exercises.

There was a catch: Tommy loves Ben & Jerry's ice cream. He ate it every single night. By no means was Tommy fat, but I thought that by removing the ice cream, we might be able to take him from 10 percent body fat down to maybe 6 or 7 percent. I also wasn't opposed to Tommy losing a little muscle, since he was already one of the strongest CrossFit athletes. If he could take 10 to 12 pounds off his frame, it meant taking an equal number off the amount of weight he'd have to lift for every single body-weight exercise. That could be a game changer in a competition where you have to do hundreds of reps.

At the end of a hard Saturday training session, I told Tommy he needed to lay off the ice cream until the CrossFit Games were over. He was bummed out, but he complied—Tommy was extremely dedicated and would do anything to win.

Over the following week, something funny happened: Tommy was slower on the rower, his IWT (interval weight training) numbers dropped across the board (you'll learn about these savage workouts later), and he wasn't as strong. At first, I thought he was just having a couple of off days. That can happen for reasons ranging from bad sleep to stress at home, but the pattern continued.

Tommy and I sat down and looked at everything in his life that had occurred over the past couple of weeks. He was sleeping normally. He was doing all of his recovery practices diligently. His life stress was low. The only change we could settle on was that missing ice cream.

I couldn't believe the words were coming out of my mouth, but I told him to go ahead and eat his pint of Ben & Jerry's every night.

The very next time Tommy came into the gym, he was back to his old self. His rows were up to speed, his performance returned to normal, and his strength workouts were solid. When he went to the CrossFit Games that year, he performed extremely well. In the years to follow, he captained the first team to ever win the CrossFit Games two years in a row.

For Tommy, ice cream was a reward for going harder. Every time he did a workout, he'd set goals for himself. If he hit those goals, he'd reward himself with a pint of ice cream. The ice cream wasn't just food—there was a psychological attachment there.

If he hadn't eaten in a way that worked for him, he probably would have failed at being so successful. Tommy's story illustrates a critical fact: You need room in your diet for the foods you love. If you never enjoy yourself, you'll be miserable, and it's extremely difficult to work hard in that state. There's an old saying that rings true: A happy athlete is a productive athlete.

MAXIMUS-APPROVED CHEATS

Viet Pham is an Iron Chef winner, Food Network Star, *Food and Wine* magazine's Best New Chef of 2011, and three-time James Beard award semifinalist. I've trained Viet for a couple years now, and he's as dedicated as they come. I've watched him transform himself from an Iron Chef to an iron body.

I love a good cheat meal, and Viet has helped me elevate my cheat meals so they taste even better, but are actually healthier. We use organic, locally sourced, high-quality ingredients, and a little of Viet's magic. Here are Viet's instructions for the three cheats that he has helped me perfect.

Burgers: Before you cook burgers on a grill, partially freeze them or dunk them in a bucket of ice-cold water. This sets the fat so that it doesn't leach out of the burger. When it comes to seasoning, substitute out a third of the salt you'd normally use for high-quality fish sauce. Fish sauce provides amino acids and glutamic acid and will make your burger more savory.

Fried chicken: To make fried chicken extra-crispy, use a 1-to-1 ratio of a high-protein flour (such as pastry or bread flour) and cornstarch. Roll the chicken in the mixture, dip it in buttermilk, and roll again in the flour mixture with spices of your choice. To cook the chicken, fill a cast-iron skillet half-full of canola oil and heat it to about 325°F. Drop the chicken in and brown it on each side (about 12 minutes of total cooking). I favor smaller pieces of chicken because they turn out crispier and require less cooking time.

Homemade butter: Homemade butter is shockingly easy to make. Take a big Mason jar and fill it halfway with organic whipping cream. Add a couple of pinches of sea salt and a marble or a clean rock. Shake the jar vigorously for about 15 minutes. First, the cream will turn into whipped cream and then, eventually, it will turn into butter. Pour out the extra buttermilk, and you'll be left with butter. If you want thicker butter, then whisk until thick.

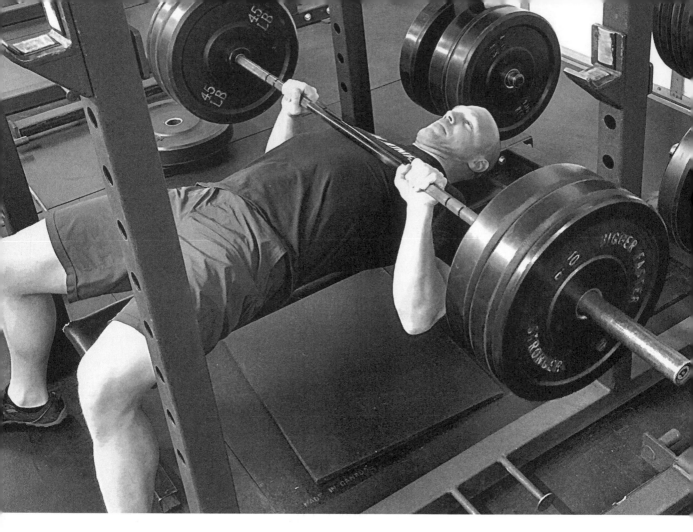

Extremely restrictive diets don't work in the long run. Life is too short to not enjoy the foods you love with the people you love. If your diet is going to work long-term, it has to be sustainable, and enjoyment is the number-one thing that will make it that way.

A smarter, more sustainable approach than saying "I'll never eat that again" is to simply make room in your diet for the foods you love. But it can't be done haphazardly: I've found that there's a specific ratio of healthy to unhealthy foods that allows you to nail any goal and also stick to your eating plan for the long haul.

FOLLOW THE MAXIMUS 90-PERCENT RULE

I searched for years for the perfect ratio of how much healthy to unhealthy food a person can eat to both enjoy himself and stick to his diet for years. I tried different healthy-food-to-unhealthy-food ratios on hundreds of different people. Time and time again, the one that works best is what I call the 90-percent rule: Eat 90 percent healthy food, and leave 10 percent for anything else you want to eat.

Eating healthy 95 percent of the time, for

example, doesn't leave enough room for enjoyment and can cause people to go off the rails. Eating healthy just 80 percent of the time is surely enjoyable and sustainable, but it allows for too large of a window for bad foods. That large window holds you back from reaching your goals.

A 90 to 10 ratio of healthy to unhealthy food is the sweet spot. It allows you to hit your goals while also eating pizza and birthday cake at your kid's party, or having a burger and a beer or two with your buddies on game day.

The beauty of this rule is that you can make it work any way you want. Let's say, for example, you eat around 2,500 calories every day. That means you could eat one roughly 250-calorie treat a day. Conversely, every 10 days, you could have one cheat day where you eat only the foods you enjoy. To prepare yourself for a food-filled Christmas Eve and day, you could eat healthy food for 18 days in a row.

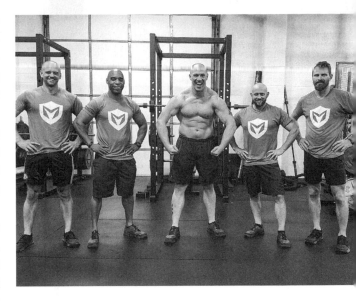

Bobby's Law:
You can't kick ass on a low-carb diet.

Be creative with your math, and figure out a way to make the 90-percent rule work for you. Do that and be accountable, and you'll build incredible fitness and enjoy doing it.

Note that there is one caveat to this rule: It only applies to your long-term diet. If you are trying to build a high level of fitness in a short period—like you will if you do The 12-Week Program on page 129—you have to be 100 percent strict 100 percent of the time. That's part of the cost, and there's no escaping it.

When you're trying to get insanely fit in an insanely short period of time, I'm sorry, but you just don't have wiggle room for pizza, burgers and fries, or beer. Commit fully, and eat strict for a handful of weeks.

That's also why you may want to consider doing a short transformation-style program at a time that's conducive to not only training hard and long every day but also to eating strictly. For example, don't do it over a time when you're going to go on vacation, or over Thanksgiving or Christmas.

14

TAKE OWNERSHIP

My nutrition rules are designed to help you figure out a method of eating that works for you. But, in reality, I consider them more akin to guidelines rather than hard-and-fast rules. Through years of working with some of the fittest, most ripped men and women on the planet, I've found that they work for most of the people, most of the time. Most people, not all people.

I, for example, can eat burgers and fries, and Tommy can eat ice cream, and it propels us to our goals. But, we both train for about 15 hours a week and are relatively large human beings. The average person just doesn't exercise enough or have the size to pull off our diets and stay lean.

Bobby's Law:
Success isn't about greatness, it is about consistency.

The best diet is always the diet that works best for you, but finding that perfect diet isn't always easy. We're constantly tempted by the next diet that promises big results. So, as you experiment and take ownership of your diet, follow these steps to make sure that your eating plan is actually the best one for you.

START WITH WHY

Jimmy Kimmel recently featured a brilliant segment. In it, a reporter walked around Los Angeles asking pedestrians whether or not they eat gluten, and why.

Gluten is a composite of proteins found in wheat, barley, and rye. About 1 or 2 percent of people suffer from celiac disease, a disease that causes their bodies to react extremely poorly to gluten. A larger number of people have gluten intolerance, which is essentially a lesser form of celiac disease. For those people, gluten causes everything from stomach issues and a foggy mind to muscle pain and rashes.

The gluten-free craze started a few years ago when people began realizing that gluten intolerance might be more prevalent than we once thought.

But, if you're not gluten-intolerant, gluten is fine for you. And if you cut it out, your diet may actually become less sustainable, since eating 100 percent gluten-free takes a lot of effort—an

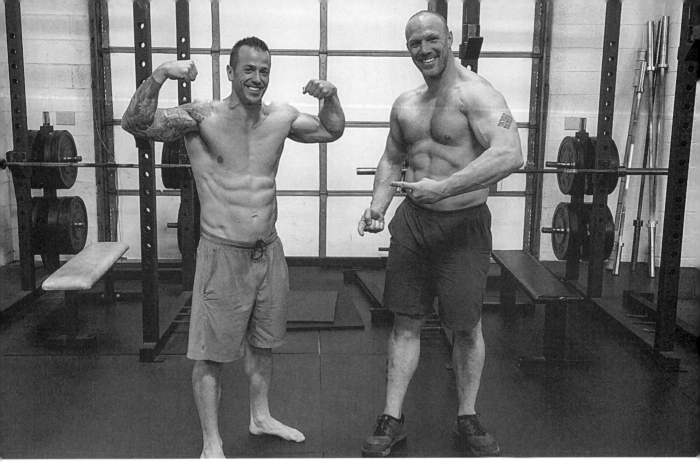

incredible number of foods contain gluten. Many people who eat gluten-free are also constantly low on muscle glycogen (your muscles' sprint fuel), so going gluten-free could even hurt your gym performance.

Somehow the gluten-free diet became the "it" thing to do, and, as Kimmel expertly put it, "So many people don't eat gluten because someone in their yoga class told them not to."

Whenever Kimmel's reporter found a person who ate gluten-free, he'd ask them what gluten is. As you might expect, they had no clue—they had answers ranging from "I don't know" to "pastries" to "wheat." They couldn't tell you what foods gluten was found in or give you a reason why they weren't eating it, other than that they heard it was "bad for you."

Don't be one of those people. Just because some guy at your gym lost 10 pounds on a gluten-free diet—or a juice fast, or by eating Paleo—doesn't mean that it's right for you. If you're interested in a particular diet, figure out why you want to try the diet.

Here's an example of a "why" that might work: "I want to go gluten-free because research shows that people with gluten intolerance often experience stomach problems and feel tired after eating gluten. Those two things happen to me after I eat wheat products. What's more, gluten intolerance runs in my family."

The answer "I don't eat gluten because my friend lost weight eating gluten-free" is not a viable response.

You'll likely have to do some research before

you have an answer that makes sense. Read some books, and do some research.

For quick information, use Wikipedia. Yes, I know it's the butt of some jokes. But a 2005 study in the journal *Nature*—the preeminent scientific journal in the world—showed that Wikipedia is just as accurate as the *Encyclopedia Britannica*.[7] And a recent study in the *Journal of Oncology Practice* found that Wikipedia had equally accurate and thorough articles about cancer as did the *Physician Data Query*.[8]

TRACK YOUR RESULTS

When a client jumps on a new eating plan, I have them track a few key points of information for a few weeks to make sure that the plan is the right fit for them. Keeping some basic records can tell you if your diet is taking your body in the direction that you want it to go.

At minimum, you should keep note of these things.

▶ **What you eat:** For at least 2 weeks, track what you're eating in a calorie-counting app. This will give you a general sense of the nutrition composition of your foods, such as how many calories and grams of carbs, fats, and proteins they have. A food scale can improve your accuracy—you'll be shocked at just how small a serving of peanut butter actually is. Once you've tracked for a couple of weeks, you should have a sense of how many calories you're eating each day, so if you eat basically the same things every day, there's no need to keep tracking.

▶ **How you feel:** This is critical. Every day, write down how you feel. Are you tired and beat down or energetic and ready to go? This can be a good gauge of whether you're eating enough. If you consistently feel tired, you might need to increase your calories, or rethink what you're eating.

▶ **How you perform:** Track your general performance numbers. If you've changed your diet in order to perform better, those figures should go up. Don't expect the improvements to come overnight. But within a month, you should see some general improvements. Conversely, cutting weight and performing better rarely go hand-in-hand. If you're trying to lose weight, the best you can do is try to keep your performance numbers where they were before you started your diet. Note that this rule does not apply if you're starting very overweight—if you're overweight and you cut pounds, you'll likely see your performance increase. It also doesn't apply to many endurance sports.

▶ **How much you weigh:** This seems like a no-brainer, but you'd be amazed at how many people don't keep tabs on their weight. Weigh yourself every day. Don't freak out if the number on the scale goes up or down a few pounds day to day—your weight fluctuates based on your hydration levels, what you eat, whether you've gone to the bathroom, and more. Write down your number each time you weigh yourself. Then, after a month or so, look to make sure that the numbers are trending in the direction you want.

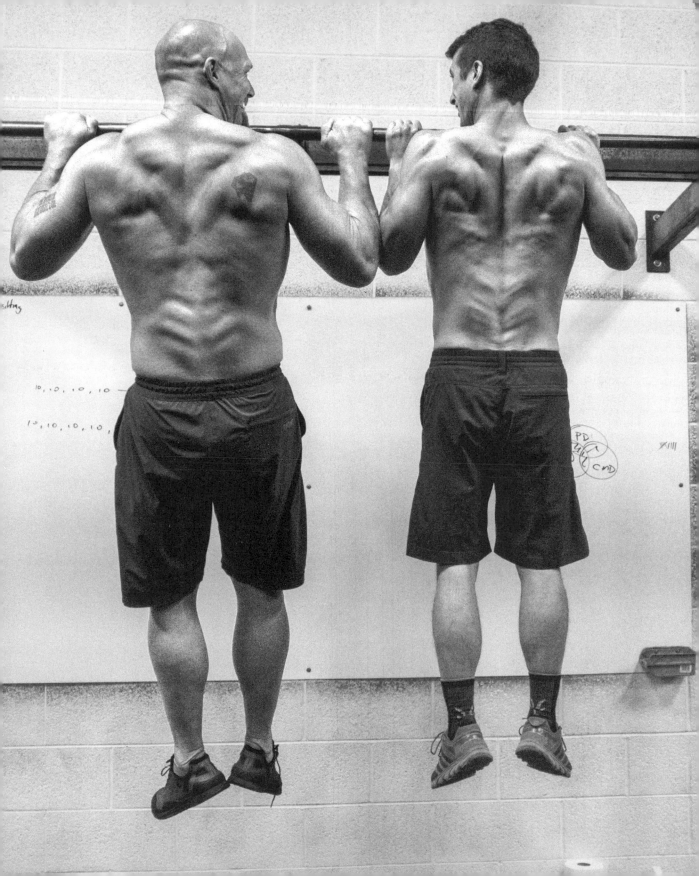

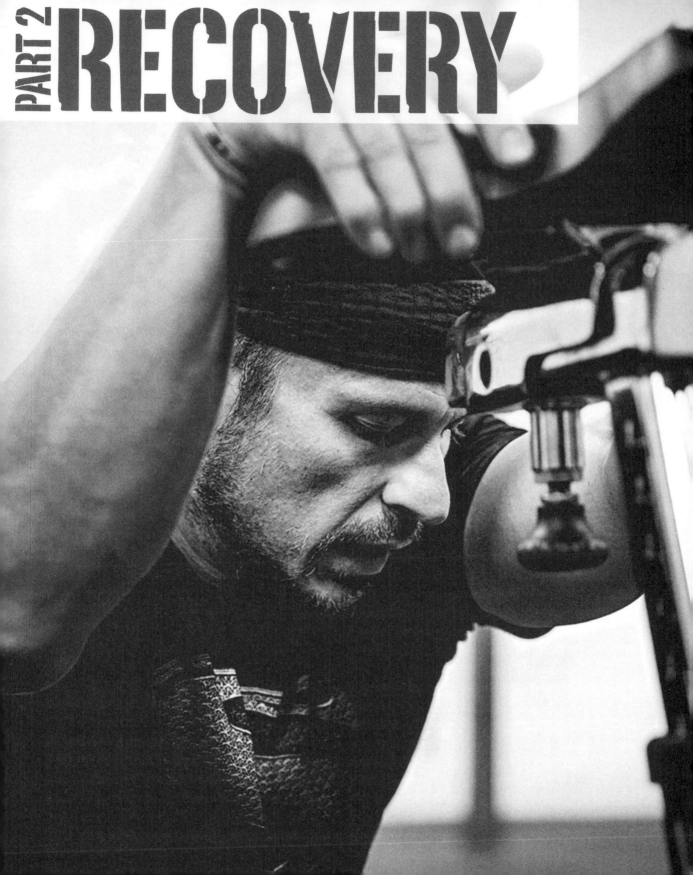

15

GET MORE SLEEP

You'd think it would be easy to compel people to do a fitness-enhancing activity that requires absolutely zero effort. But in my experience, it's the opposite. No matter if I'm working with a Hollywood actor, a professional athlete, or anyone else, even the most dedicated people struggle with sleeping enough.

The average American sleeps just 6 to 7 hours a night. I like to give everyone who works with me this analogy: Not logging enough sleep is like setting out for a long road trip with your emergency brake on. If you reach your destination, it'll have taken you much more time and energy to arrive.

Your body is no different. Leave the house with a full night's sleep, and you'll be far more productive in every facet of your life. Leave the house exhausted, and everything you do becomes more difficult and requires more time and effort.

Fitness-wise, sleep is critical, because it creates a surge of muscle-building hormones—making it one of the single best things you can do to naturally build more muscle, shed more fat, and perform better. I joke that an extra hour of sleep is like taking steroids, and magic fat-loss pills.

Science backs up my claims. Here's what a lack of sleep does to you.

▶ **It makes you more injury prone.** A University of California study found that athletes were more likely to sustain an injury when they'd slept less than 8 hours the night before.[1]

▶ **It hurts your long-term fitness.** Two studies from the Sleep Foundation analyzed the sleep habits of Major League Baseball players. They found that players who were less fatigued performed better on the field *and* had longer careers in the league.[2]

▶ **It hurts your performance.** Basketball players who logged more sleep increased their shooting accuracy by nearly 10 percent, according to scientists at Stanford University.[3]

▶ **It makes you weak.** Lifters who didn't sleep enough for a few days were significantly weaker in the bench press, leg press, and deadlift exercises compared to when they were fully rested, according to a study in the journal *Ergonomics*.[4]

▶ **It makes you slow.** Athletes on the Stanford University swim team not only swam faster, but they also exploded off the starting blocks quicker, according to research presented at the annual SLEEP conference.[5]

- **It messes with your metabolism.** Tired people experience changes in how their fat cells react, which may cause them to gain weight, according to scientists at the University of Chicago.[6]

Like all things, sleep needs can vary between people, but I've found that people who log 8 hours each night, which is how long most sleep experts recommend, tend to reach their fitness goals faster. Of course, logging 9 or 10 hours may deliver more benefits, so if you want to sleep more, you should.

When I'm working with someone who isn't hitting their sleep numbers, here are the three strategies I recommend that they use to push them to the 8-hour mark.

1. BLACK OUT YOUR BEDROOM

We evolved to sleep in the dark and to wake with the light. Darkness and light are cues that tell you when it's time to sleep and wake up. When you're asleep and light hits your skin, your body reacts like it just got a wake-up call: Your melatonin (a sleep hormone) drops and your body temperature and cortisol rise, two reactions that prime you to wake up.

Bobby's Law:
The strongest factor for your success is faith in yourself.

Back when we were living in caves, that was helpful. But in the modern world, it doesn't always make sense to wake when the sun shines through your window. What's more, electric light shining into your room can throw off your sleep pattern.

That's why I recommend that all of the people I work with install blackout curtains on their bedroom windows. These curtains only cost on average $50. But, as their name implies, they block out all outside light, whether it's the sun in the morning or a street lamp that stays on all night, allowing you to log high-quality sleep.

No, regular curtains won't do the trick. I'm talking about the kind of thick curtains you often find at nice hotels; the ones that can keep your room pitch black whether it's noon or midnight.

2. CREATE A SLEEP RITUAL

In a perfect world, you'd go to bed at 10:00 p.m. and wake up at 6:00 a.m. for work the next morning.

But in the real world, this approach rarely goes as planned. For most people, wake-up times are nonnegotiable. If you must be at work at 8:00 a.m., you either wake up early enough to arrive at work on time, or you sleep in and get fired.

The time you go to bed, on the other hand, is totally up to you. For most people, it fluctuates night to night, which impacts your long-term sleep quality.

Let's say you have to wake up at 6:00 a.m. on weekdays. Perhaps one night you decide to watch ESPN until midnight, another you become engrossed in a book and don't turn out the light until 11:30, and another night, you talk to a friend until 10:45. Now you've logged the full 8 hours of sleep you need just two out of five weeknights. Sadly, most people don't even sleep that much. I know people who are lucky to see 8 hours of sleep one night a month.

To avoid those nights where you stay up late, create a nightly sleep ritual. Once I implemented this into my own life, I was able to nix those random late nights, and I suddenly began performing better in the gym.

My family's sleep ritual typically works like this: Around 8:00 p.m., we put the kids to bed. We watch an episode of a television series until 9:00. Then, I'll usually do something to relax, like take a warm shower, use the foam roller for 20 minutes, and then read a book. Then, it's in bed with lights out by 10:00.

A few tips: Turn off your electronics 45 minutes before you go to bed. This means that you shut the TV off, put your cell phone away, and avoid scrolling through Facebook or checking e-mail. Then, do something relaxing—take a shower, read, or foam roll. You may not feel tired at first, but you need to crawl into bed and rest. It might take you a while to fall asleep, but, eventually, your body will acclimate to your new sleep routine, and you'll fall asleep on cue.

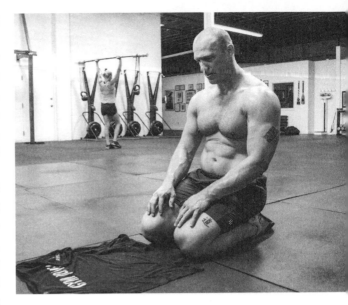

3. KEEP YOUR BEDROOM A BEDROOM

Today, too many people fill their bedrooms with all kinds of nonsense that makes it a room for a lot more than sleeping: TVs, laptops, stereos . . . the list goes on. Your bedroom is not an entertainment room or an office. Your bedroom is for two things: sleep and sex.

All of that extra stuff you bring in only distracts you from sleep. When you have a TV in your bedroom, you're likely to turn it on and stay up too late. If your laptop is in your room, you'll inevitably check and send e-mails. When you bring your phone into your bedroom, you're going to check your Instagram and text people. So get rid of the television, phone, and computer, and turn your bedroom into what it was meant to be.

What's more, research indicates that even small electronic lights can disturb your sleep patterns through the night.[7] Rid your bedroom of electronics, and you'll not only increase the quantity of your sleep, you'll also increase its quality.

16

MANAGE YOUR STRESS

A few years ago, I had a successful businessman named Len reach out and ask me to train him. He seemed dedicated and ambitious, and another person I trained with vouched for his work ethic. I agreed—I'm always happy to help someone who wants to better himself and get in shape. When I first spoke to my new client, I didn't ask him about his training history. I first asked him about his lifestyle.

He explained that he was a New York City-based financial worker who worked 80 hours a week and traveled all over the world. His job was exceedingly stressful, so much so that he only slept about 4 hours each night. His lifestyle also put a strain on his family relationships.

For the past couple of years, he'd tried to lose weight and improve his fitness, but he always failed. He bounced from trainer to trainer, and, sure, he'd seen some results, but he came nowhere close to achieving his goals.

After I heard his full story, I knew I could help him. But unfortunately, my plan wasn't what he

wanted to hear: I can help you, I said, but you're going to have to work and travel less at your current job, or you're going to have to get a new job—you need to completely overhaul your lifestyle.

This guy's stress levels were so high from work, travel, lack of sleep, and a strained personal life, that his body was using the vast majority of its resources to try to keep his stress even remotely in check. There was no program or amount of effort he could put in at the gym that could balance out the stress he was putting his body through.

Unfortunately, he wasn't willing to alter his lifestyle. I knew we'd only be spinning our wheels, so I told him I wasn't interested in training him, but to call me if he ever changed his lifestyle.

We went our separate ways, but about a year later, he called me back. He said that he'd tried a couple other trainers after we chatted and, no surprise, they couldn't deliver the results he wanted.

So, he thought I might have been on to something, and he quit his stressful job. He'd found a job he enjoyed and that didn't require him to turn over his entire life. He was wondering if I'd be willing to train him now.

I was. I wrote him a program and coached him along the way. In short order, he reached all of the goals that had been so elusive for so long.

The thing is: Regardless of whether you work 80 hours a week, spend a lot of time away from home, or have family problems, even the lowest levels of stress are a silent killer for your health and fitness.

Here's what having chronically elevated stress levels does.

▶ It raises your susceptibility to nearly every degenerative disease.

▶ It increases your risk of hypertension, heart attack, and stroke.

▶ It can cause your body to burn muscle and add unwanted body fat.

▶ It drops your testosterone and human growth hormone, sabotaging your ability to build and repair muscle.

▶ It wears down your body, making you feel tired all the time.

▶ It prevents you from recovering between work-outs.

▶ It makes you more likely to get injured and then harder to recover from those injuries.

There are two different kinds of stress: 1) eustress, a beneficial stress such as exercise, and 2) distress, a negative stress like too many hours at the office. The funny thing is that your body doesn't actually view these kinds of stress differently. It can only cope with a certain amount of stress until some-thing breaks. Each time you add stress to your body—whether it's a particularly hard workout or a fight with your significant other—it's like pouring liquid into a glass. If you keep adding liquid to the glass but never remove liquid, the glass eventually

Bobby's Law:
There are 7 days in a week. "Someday" isn't one of them.

overflows. When the glass overflows, your body throws something at you that stops you in your tracks, like sickness or an injury.

For example, researchers at the University of Missouri tracked how life stress affected their Division I college football team. The scientists found that when the players were under a high load of life stress (during testing weeks), they were twice as likely to get injured on the field.[8] Think about that: Fretting about a test made these young, fit football players more likely to blow an ACL in their knees.

Some life stress is inevitable. If your boss, for example, drops into your office and tells you that he needs a project a week earlier than the date you initially agreed upon, there's not much you can do about that. The same goes with stress that arises from random life events, like your kid being sent to the principal's office, a traffic jam, or a flat tire.

Other life stress can be avoided. Maybe you're in a bad relationship or a job that consistently asks too much of you. The key to managing stress is to take action to keep it low—keep the liquid in your glass low, so to speak. I use the following two strat-egies with everyone who trains with me. I can tell you this: The people with the least liquid in their glasses also make the most fitness gains.

CHANGE WHAT YOU CAN

There are two primary, insidious-yet-changeable stressors that I see pop up in many of my clients'

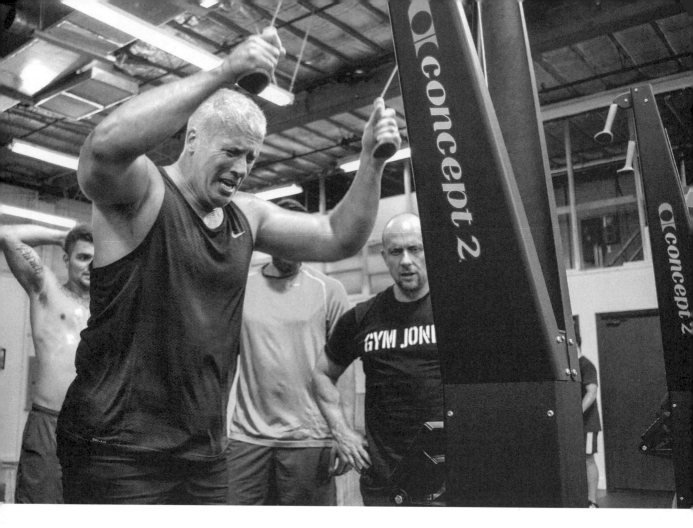

lives, filling their glasses and sucking away their happiness.

The first is working too many hours at a job that you don't like. It's basically impossible to be happy and stress-free when you're doing something you hate, in a place you hate, for more than half of your waking hours, according to people I've talked to in that situation. The stress hurts everything you can do, fitness-wise. More important, it degrades your overall quality of life: People who are miserable at work are miserable overall.

Job descriptions rarely change. Once your employer has an expectation that you'll work a lot of hours, they're not going to be happy if you sud-

denly cut back and work less. But your quality of life is on the line: If you need to work less, have a conversation about it with your employer. Hopefully, they'll work with you to alter your schedule and the duties of your job. Chances are, if you're happier and less stressed, you'll still be able to deliver to them what they need. If that doesn't work, I strongly suggest that you find a new job.

That's a frightening proposition, yes, but I've never met anyone who's done this who regretted it. Take my friend Jay Collins.

In 2011, Jay was working as a New Hampshire-based mortgage broker. He worked well over 50 hours a week, was under a tremendous amount of stress, and he hated the work that he did. In short, he was miserable. Jay's family relationships were strained, his health was suffering, and he was depressed.

Jay had recently started training a few coworkers for fun, and it dawned on him that helping people reach fitness goals was his passion. He decided that he wanted to open his own gym, and he had two amazing things going for him: a wife who believed in him and a work ethic second to none. He was terrified to quit his job, like most people are, but he finally reached a tipping point and left.

He didn't have a bunch of money stored away in the bank. He had desperation, and for Jay, that was enough.

It was terrifying, of course. Jay had children in college, and his entire family was accustomed to a comfortable lifestyle. But knowing that he simply couldn't fail compelled him to work his ass off to build that gym and make it successful.

Nine months after quitting, Jay opened his own private gym, and now, MaxEdge Fitness Training in Hampton, New Hampshire, has more than 300 members and is one of the most successful private gyms in the northeastern United States. What's more, his relationships with his wife and kids have improved exponentially.

Bobby's Law:
It costs nothing to be nice.

I'm not suggesting that you quit your job today and figure out your plan later. It's helpful to save money to make a life transition easier. But, there are people who transform their lives without a safety net every single day. Don't be too afraid to make big changes in the name of self-improvement.

The second big pitfall is a bad relationship. I'll be the first to admit that I've been in a relationship that lasted more than a year that should have lasted no more than a week. In a bad relationship, you expend far too much effort fighting, arguing, and trying to make it work, when it never will. It's like running on a treadmill: You'll put in lots of effort without actually getting anywhere.

It's amazing how often relationship issues are the root of a short-term fitness problem. But, when we're in a bad romantic situation, it's easy to put blinders on. Here are some of the most common signs.

▶ You're always critical of each other.

▶ You don't trust each other.

▶ You fight all the time.

▶ Your friends avoid hanging out with you if you're bringing your significant other.

It's easy to become dependent on the other person, and to be scared to cut the cord and be single again.

But my advice is to cut the cord as soon as you can. Don't waste your time and energy fighting a losing battle. Yes, you might be sad for a week, or even a month. But, after the initial shock and wave of emotions pass, you'll soon be far less stressed and also happier. Soon, you'll wonder why you didn't bail earlier.

No one ever regrets leaving a bad relationship—myself included.

DE-STRESS EVERY DAY

The best way to deal with general, unpreventable life stress—work projects, misbehaving kids, or accidents—is to find a daily way to cope.

Most experts agree that spending 10 to 20 minutes each day doing something that reduces your stress can positively affect your long-term fitness and health. This can help you recover faster, avoid injury and sickness, and boost your happiness, according to a wide body of research reported by the American Psychological Association.

A few years ago, a good friend of mine asked me if I meditate. I laughed and told him to stop being ridiculous. Then, I actually gave it some thought. I don't meditate in the traditional sense of the word, but I do take a 20- to 30-minute walk after lunch every single day. On my walk, I completely disconnect from the outside world—I don't check my phone, and I don't think about my work or my day-to-day problems—I just clear my thoughts and relax. I suppose it's my own form of meditation, because on the days I don't take my walk, I feel more uptight. If I don't take that walk for a few days in a row, I feel scattered and like I don't have as much energy.

Your method of dealing with stress can be anything that works for you. I know people who de-stress by meditating, using coloring books, reading, building Lego sets, and woodworking.

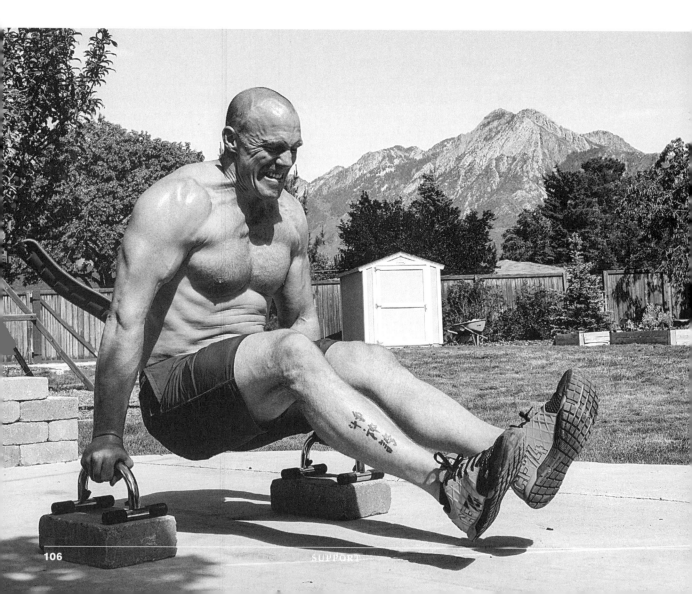

SUPPORT

17

LISTEN TO YOUR BODY

Jason Archibald is one of the most dedicated athletes I work with. He trains with me 5 days a week, often coming into the gym twice a day.

Recently, we did a training session filled with box jumps and squats—two moves that build explosive power and athleticism. As we began the workout, everyone could see that Jason wasn't producing his usual strength and power.

He said he felt fine, so we continued adding more weight to the bar and using successively higher boxes for the jumps. Then things went wrong. Jason lined up to attempt his highest box jump of the day, missed, and sliced both his shins open on the box.

"I knew I shouldn't have been jumping today," Jason said. "I didn't sleep well the past few nights, and I felt weak coming into the gym today."

Jason's story illustrates a phenomenon I see often. People often become married to a training program, and believe it's written in stone—as if doing bench press as it's programmed on Monday makes it infinitely more effective than doing it on Tuesday. Or, people make some progress, love the feeling, and think that if they take it easy, they'll lose all their gains.

If you train 5 days a week, you'll log 260 workouts in a year. Taking a recovery day when you feel beat down is not going to derail your fitness. In fact, it might actually improve it. That's because not feeling "quite right," or having aches and pains, is your body's way of telling you that something is wrong, and that you may need to back off. Let's analyze each issue.

NOT FEELING QUITE RIGHT

Every day, I have a group of people—ranging from average guys to pro athletes—that meet me in the gym at 9:00 a.m. for an hour- or 2-hour-long training session. We reconvene at 4:00 p.m. for another difficult workout.

When the people I train feel beat down or tired, it's usually because they're not doing the recovery practices you'll learn next, or they're not eating enough.

Training as much as we do requires a lot of energy. If I had to guess, I'd say that we each burn, on average, an extra 1,000 to 2,000 calories a day through exercise. There are workouts in this book that likely burn 1,000 calories each, like IWTs and long endurance sessions (you'll learn more about these in Section V: The Maximus Manual on page 149).

Once you add a significant amount of exercise into your life, your energy needs go up. If you're trying to lose weight, burning more total calories than you take in—through living and exercise—is how you lose weight. But if you're trying to increase your performance or gain weight, you need to eat the amount of calories you're burning or more. It's simple supply and demand.

Eating less than you burn causes you to run at a deficit. You essentially start digging a hole, and your body begins to use muscle along with fat as fuel. That sinks your performance and causes you to feel bad.

Bobby's Law:
Don't go around obstacles. Go right through them.

When this happens, I'll often sit down with my clients and analyze and tweak their eating plans, adding in a few hundred calories at first, and then have them double down on their recovery practices.

Or you just may need to take it easy for a couple days. If a client is worn down, we still train, but their area of focus changes. They might do an easy cardiovascular workout, like rowing slowly for an hour. Or they'll work on their exercise form with light weights, or do corrective exercises. Either way, they'll log valuable work that adds to their overall levels of fitness without harm.

ACHES AND PAINS

Aches, pains, and injuries can also indicate that something is off-balance with your training or your recovery status.

Recently, a few friends and I went to a park near the gym to do an outdoor workout. The training included lunging and sprinting. Everyone in the crew had a long training history and was supremely fit. But one of the guys, just 10 minutes into the workout, pulled his hamstring. His problem: He was neglecting injury-proofing exercises.

Aches and pains are a sign that you're not recovering properly, or that you're neglecting injury-proofing exercises. A huge part of recovery isn't just bringing your body back to normalcy, it's doing work that allows you to prevent and avoid injuries.

First, always be flexible with your training program. You don't get fit in just one workout—it's training session after session after session where the benefits stack up and you see a difference. Never power through pain. If your knees hurt, for example, don't do your lower body that day—do upper-body work. If your shoulder hurts, lay off the overhead presses and focus on your lower body. If your back hurts, don't do deadlifts. It's a pretty simple concept.

You also need to take the time to identify the reasons that you may feel certain aches and pains in the first place. Then, you have to work to fix them. This may include warming up the right way, doing supplemental work, paying attention to form, and also doing extra "physiotherapy" exercises outside the gym.

The following are the most common pains I

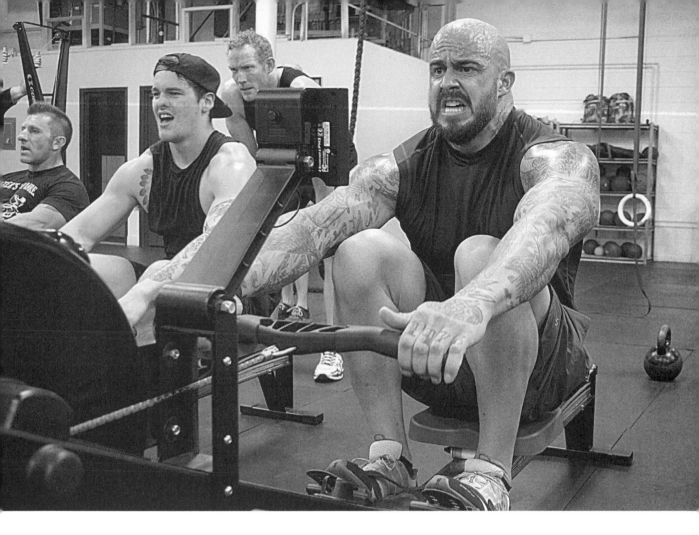

see and the methods that I find most often correct them. Of course, if you have a pain, you should first see a doctor, who may refer you to a physical therapist. By no means is this list set in stone or exhaustive—I'm just laying out why the following issues happen to most people, and the most common solution for each.

Knee Pain

Knee pain often stems from having weak hips. When your hips are weak, you can't stabilize your knees, which causes them to go out of alignment when you run, jump, and do lower-body exercises. That sends force to your delicate joints instead of

your muscles, which can lead to injury. To fortify your hips, do exercises that involve a hip-thrusting motion. I like deadlifts, hip thrusts with a barbell, and jump squats.

Shoulder Pain

Your form is probably bad when you bench press and do overhead lifts. This causes the weight to shift to your small rotator cuff muscles, which creates pain and leads to injury. Fix this two ways. First, strengthen your rotator cuff muscles. Do external rotation exercises while you lie on the couch each night (use a 5-pound weight). Second, fix your form on your overhead lifts and bench

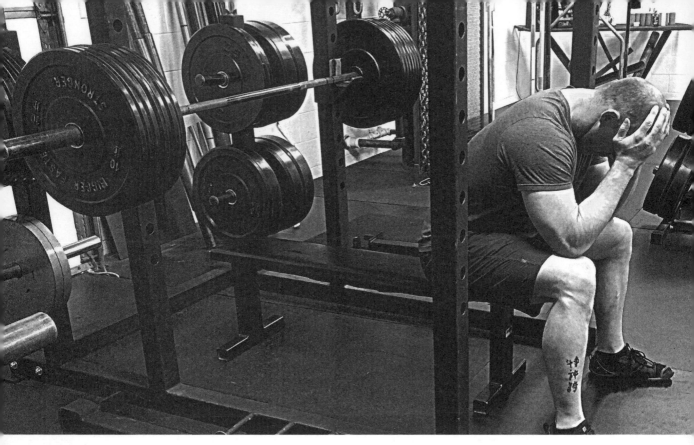

Talk minus action equals zero.

press. While your pain heals, lay off those lifts. Regardless of whether your shoulder hurts or not, pay particularly close attention to your form when you lift weights with your arm in the "high-five" position (exercises such as shoulder presses or upright rows). Research shows that those exercises are most likely to set you up for injury (see page 240 for the proper form to use when doing an overhead press).

Hip Pain

Tight muscles typically cause hip pain. When your hips are tight—this usually occurs mostly on your left side—it can throw off their alignment, shifting weight to small muscles and inducing pain. The fix is easy: Stretch your hips at night when you watch TV. I typically include the "Modified Pigeon" (see page 113). Stretch your left side more than your right.

Low-Back Pain

Your core is likely too weak to "lock down" your spine and keep it straight when you do exercises like kettlebell swings and deadlifts (bending your spine and using improper form under load is what leads to injuries like a bulged disk and induces pain). So do four key core exercises a few times a week: cat camels, curlups, bird dogs, and side planks. Researchers from the University of Waterloo say that these four moves are the best way to bolster your core and protect your spine.[9]

PRACTICE YOUR RECOVERY

I never use the words "rest day" when I write a program, and there's a good reason for that.

I've had a handful of clients come to me with this story: They arrive in decent shape, but just can't seem to reach the next level. We first look at their nutrition, and it's generally pretty close to what I'd recommend. Then, we look at their training programs. They, too, are in good shape, including five weekly workouts. But, typically, the two other days will only list one word: "Rest."

"What do you do on your rest days?" I'll ask.

"Literally, nothing, because it's a rest day," the person usually says with a laugh. "I sit all day at work and then go home and watch Netflix."

A lot of people look at their rest days as an excuse to be a vegetable. But, that actually sets you back, because prolonged sitting and lying reduces blood flow to your muscles, hurting your ability to recover. It also impacts your mobility, so you'll be stiffer and may not be able to work as hard on your training days, or will be more likely to sustain an injury.

My fix for these people is straightforward: First, I let them know that there are no "rest days." There are only "recovery days." Then, I give them a list of the following recovery practices, and require that they perform at least two of them on each recovery day.

Look at it this way: I work with people anywhere from 3 to 10 hours a week. Even a person who spends 10 hours a week with me is only giving me 6 percent of his time. In the 94 percent of his remaining time, he can either improve or mess everything up by being lazy or engaging in behaviors that aren't conducive to a high level of fitness.

What separates people who reach their goals quickly and those who struggle often comes down to what they're willing to do in the hours that they aren't in the gym.

So, start thinking of your rest days as recovery days. Recovery includes rest, of course, but, by definition, it means to restore yourself to a state of normalcy, and that takes action.

It's amazing how quickly people improve when they add a couple recovery practices into days they used to be a complete vegetable. Attention to recovery is often the factor that pushes people to finally attain their goals, no matter if it's to lose more weight or to lift more weight.

Below is a list of recovery practices, listed by how often you should do them. Carry out at least one of these on training days, and two on recovery days, and I can guarantee that you'll not only get closer to your goal, you'll get there faster and will feel better every day.

FOAM ROLL

Just by living your daily life and exercising, some of your muscle groups become tighter than others. That's a problem, because exercising when you have overly tight areas throws you out of balance and increases your risk of injury. Tight muscles can prevent you from getting into the correct form in an exercise, which shifts the weight to vulnerable areas.

For example, if your hips and ankles are tight—two issues that are common if you sit often—you

If plan A doesn't work, there are 25 other letters in the alphabet.

won't be able to squat with correct form. Your torso will tip forward to compensate, and the weight will shift to your delicate low back instead of your hips and legs.

Foam rolling—where you "steam roll" your muscles with a foam roller or PVC pipe—helps free tension on your muscles, allowing you to move better. In fact, researchers in Canada found that foam rolling increased study participants' mobility by 16 percent. Just 2 minutes of rolling before a workout did the trick.[10] Target a tight area that you're about to work—if you're squatting, for example, roll your hips and quads.

Outside of the gym, I recommend that you foam roll for 5 to 10 minutes each night as you wind down for the evening. The best way to do this is to roll as you watch TV. Roll over all your muscles, focusing in on your calves, hamstrings, quads,

YOU CAN'T OVERRECOVER

I have a lot of clients who go all-in with their training. The thing is that they rarely attack their recovery with the same vigor. Colin Kubarych is not one of those people.

Colin, a rock climber, came to train with me to completely overhaul his fitness. He had 3 months that he could spend with us. I wasn't sure that he'd last even 3 days—he had a lot of imbalances, lacked horsepower, and was completely in over his head. I told him that if he was going survive the training, he'd need to pay attention to recovery.

He worked hard in the gym, of course, but he didn't just pay attention to recovery, he went absolutely nuts with it. He lived on a foam roller. He slept 10 hours a night. He did contrast showers and took ice baths after every workout. He spent at least an hour a day doing structural, or rehab, work so he'd avoid injury. He walked to and from the gym.

The result: Colin made the fastest transformation I've seen in my entire career. His fitness improved so much that I made him a Gym Jones fully certified instructor.

I'm not saying that you need to go as crazy as Colin did, but I am saying that the more recovery practices you do, the quicker you'll reach your goal.

glutes, back, and shoulders. This is especially critical after a hard training bout, because it might also help reduce postworkout soreness, according to more research from Canada.[11]

For a more intense effect, you can even roll your tight spots with a lacrosse ball. Really dig in, paying special attention to your glutes and shoulders.

MOBILIZE

Foam rolling isn't the only way to mobilize your joints so that you can use better form before a workout.

Most guys don't stretch before a workout, and if they do, it's a handful of seemingly random stretches like toe touches or butt kicks. Stretching areas at random may not actually help you, because the muscles you're targeting may not even be tight in the first place. The better way is to directly target your tightest areas with a handful of mobility drills.

It turns out that no one is unique when it comes to muscle imbalances. Most people have the same tight areas, and that's because so many people sit for the majority of the day—at work, in their cars, or while watching TV.

Taking just a few minutes to do a few drills before a workout will allow you to use better form while working out, and, over time, you'll begin to move better and get more out of your fitness. In fact, not being able to move well holds back your fitness, because you'll have to use more energy to use correct form.

I have a friend who never focused on his mobility, assuming he was better off cramming more lifting into his hour at the gym. When he finally got injured from years of less-than-perfect form, he devoted just 10 minutes before each workout to improving his movement. He used the mobility exercises listed below, which were recommended to him by a doctor of physical therapy and special forces soldier named Doug Kechijian, DPT.

The result: He not only alleviated his pain, he also was able to put his body into positions he never had before, like a deep squat. That ability to go through a greater range of motion in each exercise allowed him to work muscles in ways that he hadn't before, and his performance exploded. Within a few months, he'd doubled his pushup and pullup numbers and was running 1.5 miles in less than 9 minutes, with ease. His body reacted to that newfound fitness by shedding fat and adding muscle.

These are the stretches he did, and they're incredibly helpful for most people, so try folding them into your routine. Chances are that they'll mobilize your tightest areas and help you, too, obtain serious performance gains.

Lat Hang

This exercise loosens the muscles that run down the sides of your back, allowing you to better lift overhead, avoiding upper-body problems.

Hang from a pullup bar with your feet on a bench so your knees and hips are each bent about 90 degrees. Flex your hamstrings and glutes so that your pelvis is slightly tilted up. Maintain that position throughout. Take a big breath in, then blow all the air out, as if it's toxic. You should feel a stretch in the muscles under your armpits. Take 10 big breaths while hanging.

Modified Pigeon

Most guys tend to be tightest in their left side hip. That imbalance throws your hips off-center and can cause problems ranging from hip to knee to back pain. This stretch reduces that left-side tension and centers your hips.

Get down on all fours and place a pillow or

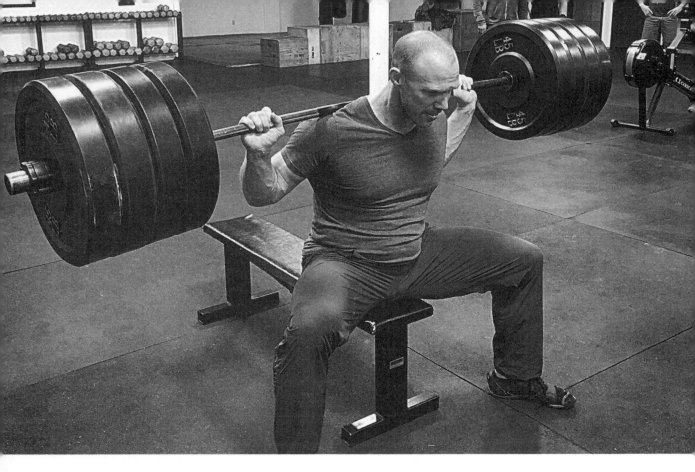

foam roller under your left knee. Lift your right knee and place it behind and to the left of your left calf. Rock your hips side to side for 2 minutes. You should feel your left hip stretch.

Couch Stretch

This stretch opens up your hips and quads, helping you to perform better in most lower-body and endurance exercises.

Assume a kneeling position, with your right foot on the floor and your knee bent 90 degrees. Place the front of your left shin up against a vertical surface, like a box, wall, or couch. You may need to hold on to something at first. Hold the position for 1 to 2 minutes as you contract the stretched leg's hamstring. Repeat with your right leg.

Deep Squat

Squatting is the most athletic exercise. This drill loosens your hips and low back, so you can achieve good squat form.

With your feet shoulder-width apart, push your knees forward and then squat as low as you can until your butt is just above the floor (you might have to hold light dumbbells in your hands to achieve this position). Hold the position, and take five long, deep breaths. Stand back up.

WALK

I've been training since I was in high school. My fitness is rather high, so when I improve, it's usually in very small doses. But a few years back, I saw a quick jump in my strength and endurance levels—I was lifting more and running faster. I hadn't experienced significant fitness gains in years.

I analyzed what I'd changed, and when I found the answer, I was shocked. I'd recently adopted a dog, and I was walking the dog for 30 to 60 minutes every day.

Many people in the fitness world bash walking as too mellow to do any good for your fitness. Yes, if you're only walking, you're probably not going to get that fit. But, I've found that a daily walk can actually be hugely beneficial for people who train hard. It pumps blood through your system, which flushes your muscles. That helps you recover from tough workouts and is a low-impact way to slightly improve your endurance and burn some calories.

Take a 30-minute stroll every day, or at least a few days a week. You could do this first thing in the morning, on your lunch break at work, or right after dinner.

My favorite way to do this is to leave my cell phone at home and just totally disconnect from the world. This makes walking a part of both my recovery and relaxation practice. Often, my wife will join the dog and me. Having 30 minutes together where we're forced to talk—with no cell phones or technology around—is a great way to improve our recovery and communication.

MASSAGE

A massage works on the same principle as foam rolling. In fact, think of it like a longer, more-effective and targeted foam-rolling session. It can restructure your muscles so that you move better and recover quicker.

The key here is to find a good sports massage therapist. He or she will likely tailor their approach to your current training program. For example, my massage therapist can feel my hamstrings and immediately know that I've been doing a lot of box jumps lately. Then, he'll tell me to lay off for a bit so I don't get injured.

When people ask me how often they should get a massage, my answer is straightforward, but a little vague: as often as you can. Massage can be expensive, averaging about $100 for an hour. I get one about once a week and see a huge benefit from it. If money is tight, I think you can get away with one a month, although two a month would be better.

CONTRAST SHOWERS

After a tough workout, your muscles fill with metabolic by-products. Taking a shower where you go from hot to cold water makes your blood vessels expand then contract, which increases blood flow and flushes those by-products, speeding recovery. Get in a shower and cook in the warm water for 3 to 5 minutes. Then, turn the water to cold and stand in it for another 3 to 5 minutes. Do that a time or two more.

ICE BATHS

If you want to avoid soreness after a race or a grueling workout, learn to love the cold. The science on whether ice baths are beneficial in the long run is mixed, but the number of anecdotes from athletes who claim ice baths help them recover quicker is overwhelming—ice baths limit muscle soreness, and also reduce your body temperature after a very difficult workout, potentially speeding recovery. Place 30 to 50 pounds of ice in the bathtub, and fill it with cold water. Sit in the water for 10 to 15 minutes. The water doesn't need to be overly cold. Anything lower than 42 degrees is overkill.

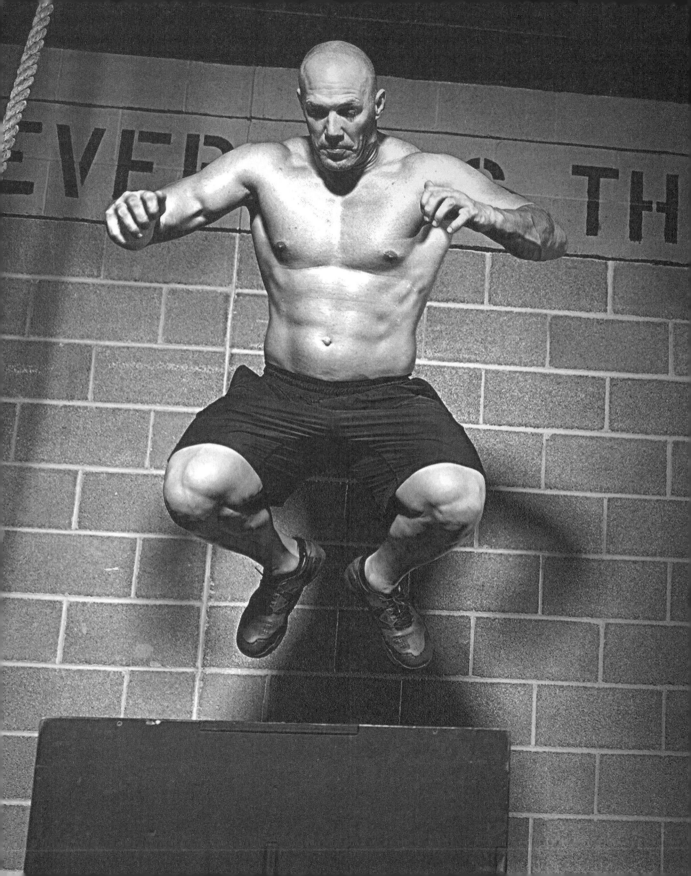

THE
MAXIMUS
METHOD

There are a lot of programs out there that promise six-pack abs and superhero fitness by working out in as little as 20 minutes a day for just 3 weeks.

This is not one of those programs.

It works off the universal truth that "there is no such thing as a free lunch." It doesn't matter if you're 25, 45, or 65, you can't reach real fitness training with just a handful of minutes a week. If you want to see the fitness results you desire, you're going to have to work your ass off for it.

Dive in. Sweat. Be sore. Feel some discomfort. You won't regret it.

In Section I: Psychology, you learned about the 130-hour rule (see page 37). Its premise is simple: For most people, it takes about 130 hours of hard work spread across 6 months to become fit.

That equates to training approximately an hour a day, 5 days a week, for 6 months straight. There are no shortcuts. You can't train just 3 hours a week and expect the same result. But if you make a strong commitment—put in the time, work hard, eat right, and recover well—I can guarantee you'll succeed.

The following section contains the 6-month training program I give anyone who wants to radically improve their fitness, body, and mind. The program is completely manageable. I know that 5 hours of weekly training, and some ancillary time and attention to nutrition and recovery, is doable for anyone—I've seen extremely busy family men and women who work 70 hours a week succeed with this program. To give you some perspective, 5 hours is just under 3 percent of your week. If you can't commit 3 percent of your life to your health and fitness, you don't really want to improve. It's that simple.

I designed this program so that you can repeat it for as long as you want. It's a sustainable fitness program that you could theoretically do for decades to come.

The 6-month program is my go-to for most people. But, some people come to me and complain that 6 months is just too long to wait. Perhaps they have a wedding or a reunion, an upcoming big-screen role, or a big competition that they want to be in shape for. There is another way.

I give those people The 12-Week Program (see page 129). I've witnessed actors, professional athletes, and everyday people make truly remarkable transformations in less than 3 months by following this program.

In it, you won't work any less than you would in my 6-month program. The 130-hour rule still stands, but you'll be forced to pack your hours into half the time.

The 12-week program requires that you train 11 hours each week. That equates to two 1-hour workouts a day, 5 days a week, and 1 day where you do just one workout. But the cost doesn't stop there. The shorter program also requires more dedication to your nutrition and recovery. You'll need to monitor calories and make sure every meal is on point, sleep 8 to 9 hours each night, do recovery practices every day, and keep your life low stress.

The good news is that you're allowed one full recovery day each week. Trust me, you'll need it.

Fair warning: The 12-week program isn't easy. It requires a serious commitment. You'll likely have to rearrange parts of your life and make sacrifices. You'll suffer. You'll face moments where you want to quit. But along the way, you'll become fitter than you ever thought possible, and you'll totally transform your body. You'll also learn something about yourself: That you're more capable than you ever imagined.

Whichever program or whatever path you choose, fully commit. Don't do anything half-assed.

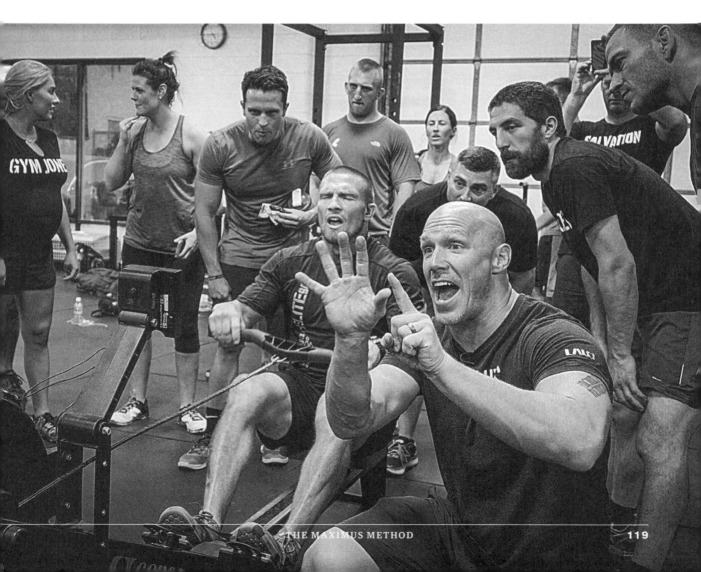

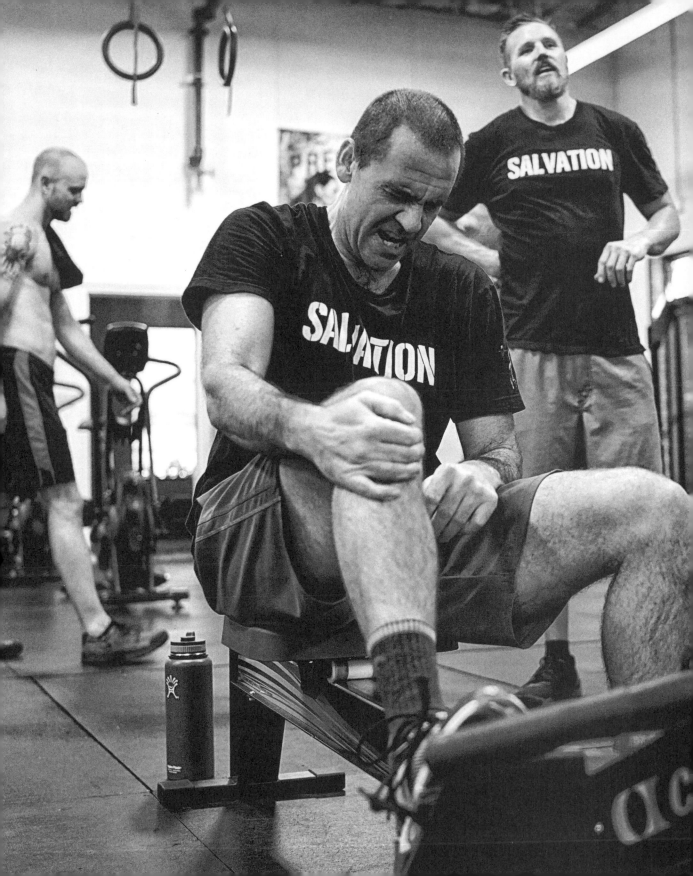

THE 6-MONTH PROGRAM

The 6-month program is broken down into six 1-month blocks. Each 4-week block gives you 1 week of training. So, you'll repeat that week for 4 weeks, then move on to the next block. Each block focuses on building a specific aspect of your fitness. This increases your overall fitness better than if you were to try to train all fitness skills equally at once, a notion I've always preached and was recently confirmed by a study in the *Journal of Strength and Conditioning Research*.[1]

This program might be less time-intensive compared to the 12-week program, but your hours must be well-spent: When you're exercising, work your ass off. And, of course, follow my nutrition and recovery rules along the way.

I won't tell you exactly what workout you should do each day. Instead, I've designed this program in a way that allows you to choose from a short list of workouts. I designed it that way for a few reasons. First, you'll learn more about exercise and will become more accountable for your own fitness. Second, it allows you to make swaps and substitutions based on your strengths and weaknesses, the equipment you have on hand, and your life schedule. Ultimately, it makes the program more enjoyable.

HOW IT WORKS

Each block includes 1 week of training that you'll repeat for 4 weeks. Each day of a training block lists the workout formats you'll do that day. To build your whole workout, you'll go to the Maximus Manual, select one of each listed format, then perform each as instructed. So, for example, if you look at the template for Block 1, Tuesday's training session calls for the following: Warmup, Challenge, Finisher, Cooldown.

To build your custom training session that day, you'll flip back to Section V: The Maximus Manual, beginning on page 149. You'll first go to the warmup section and select a warmup. Then, you'll go to the "IX: Challenges" section (page 205) and select a workout. Next, you'll go to the Finishers starting on page 219 and select one. Finally, you will complete a cooldown in Cooldowns on page 233, concluding the day.

Using the previous example, I created the following sample training session.

Warmup
Warmup 2: Total Body

Challenge
Challenge 1: 2K Row

Finisher
Finisher 8: Pushup Maximus

Cooldown
Cooldown 2: The Standard

GUIDELINES

As you go through the program, these guidelines will boost your success.

1. Address your weaknesses.

A weakness in one realm of fitness holds back your ability to improve in all the others. Fix it, and you'll see better results across the board. When you're choosing a workout, err on the side of selecting one that includes an exercise you're not good at. If, for

example, you struggle at rowing, and the workout allows you to choose between multiple cardio machines, you should choose the rower.

2. Don't always do the same workouts.

There is nothing wrong with repeating a few of your favorite workouts week to week, but make sure that you're including as much variety as possible. This ensures that you're working your body and improving your fitness skills in balance, helping you see better results.

3. Choose a warmup that complements your workout.

Your warmup should prime the area you're about to work. If, for example, your workout involves a lot of lower-body exercises, you should pick a warmup that targets your lower body. This allows you to perform better in your workout, and, therefore, improve your fitness to a greater degree.

4. Choose a finisher that's opposite of your workout.

My simple rule of thumb: If I lifted weights in my workout, my finisher is cardiovascular in nature. If

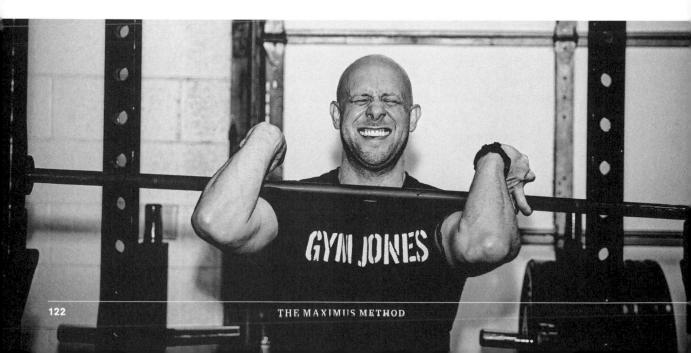

my workout taxed my cardiovascular system, I do a finisher that addresses strength. This approach leads to a more holistic workout, and better long-term results.

5. Don't be afraid to substitute days and workouts.

There will come times when you can't do the workout listed on the day listed. If you're supposed to do a workout on Tuesday, but it's just not possible that day, it's okay to rearrange your days and do your workouts on other days of the week. Or, perhaps you don't have access to equipment one day, or something comes up that cuts your time short. You can substitute other workouts. I've included 16 no-gear workouts (see page 190) for these moments. You can do them anywhere, anytime—just do them fast and hard.

6. Do an occasional weekend workout.

This program is based on 1 hour of training a day, 5 days a week, for 24 weeks. Do the math, and that only adds up to 120 hours. To make up the balance and fulfill your 130-hour requirement, you'll need to do an occasional workout on the weekend. Those are included in the programs.

7. Have fun.

Exercise shouldn't feel like a punishment. Take measures to make your workout fun, whether it's investing in the right headphones and music, setting micro-goals for yourself, or just rewarding yourself with an amazing cheat meal each week. If you don't enjoy your program, it will be harder than it needs to be. Appreciate the journey, and don't stress about the end results . . . they will come.

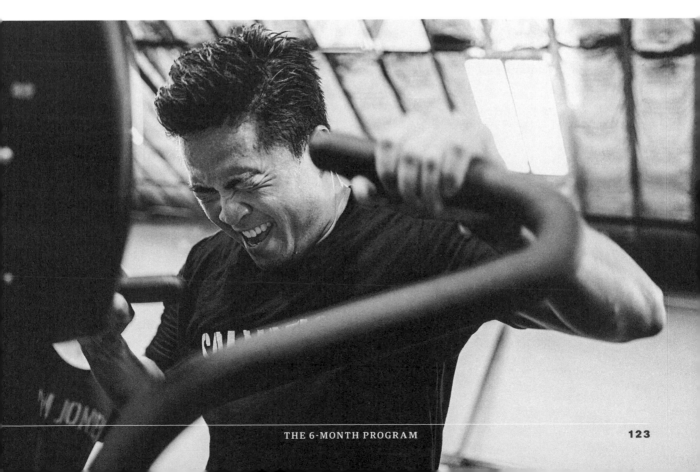

THE PROGRAM

BLOCK 1
WEEKS 1 TO 4

In the first block of this program, you'll build a baseline of general fitness and test yourself to evaluate your strengths and weaknesses. You'll figure out key numbers you need to know to get the most from the next blocks of training. What's more, you'll also find your limits, so you can smash through them.

When you do the "Max Tests" (see page 159) workouts, make sure that you perform each of the max tests, including the barbell bench press, barbell overhead press, barbell deadlift, barbell front squat, barbell back squat, and barbell overhead squat. Once you've determined your numbers on all of the max tests, you can do challenge workouts on days that call for max tests.

Monday: Warmup, Max Test, Finisher, Cooldown

Tuesday: Warmup, Challenge, Finisher, Cooldown

Wednesday: Warmup, Max Test or Challenge, Finisher, Cooldown

Thursday: Warmup, Challenge, Finisher, Cooldown

Friday: Warmup, Challenge, Finisher, Cooldown

Saturday: Rest or Recovery (Cardiovascular)

Sunday: Rest or Recovery (Cardiovascular)

BLOCK 2
WEEKS 5 TO 8

This is where the real training begins—prepare to breathe hard and heavy. Block 2 focuses on increasing your cardiovascular fitness, so you'll be able to tolerate the increasingly difficult work to come. The better your cardiovascular fitness, the more work you'll be able to do not only when you work out, but also when you have to do any physical task in everyday life. What's more, this training will also help you recover quicker and more fully during and between subsequent workouts.

Monday: Warmup, Circuit-Style, Finisher, Cooldown

Tuesday: Warmup, Interval, Finisher, Cooldown

Wednesday: Warmup, IWT, Finisher, Cooldown

Thursday: Warmup, Time Trial, Cooldown

Friday: Warmup, Circuit-Style, Finisher, Cooldown

Saturday: Rest or Warmup, Interval, Finisher, Cooldown

Sunday: Rest or Recovery (Cardiovascular)

BLOCK 3

WEEKS 9 TO 12

Now that you've laid a solid foundation of cardiovascular efficiency, you're going to build some serious horsepower. In this block, you'll attain an incredibly high level of strength and power.

Monday: Warmup, Strength and Power, Finisher, Cooldown

Tuesday: Warmup, Interval, Finisher, Cooldown

Wednesday: Warmup, Strength and Power, Finisher, Cooldown

Thursday: Warmup, Time Trial, Cooldown

Friday: Warmup, Circuit-Style, Finisher, Cooldown

Saturday: Rest or Recovery (Weighted)

Sunday: Rest or Recovery (Cardiovascular)

BLOCK 4

WEEKS 13 TO 16

This block focuses on trading your body fat for muscle. Having more useful muscle and less fat on your frame not only makes you look better but also helps your body tolerate hard work, improving your fitness.

Monday: Warmup, Mass Gain, Finisher, Cooldown

Tuesday: Warmup, Time Trial, Cooldown

Wednesday: Warmup, Mass Gain, Finisher, Cooldown

Thursday: Warmup, Interval, Finisher, Cooldown

Friday: Warmup, IWT, Finisher, Cooldown

Saturday: Rest or Recovery (Weighted)

Sunday: Rest or Recovery (Cardiovascular)

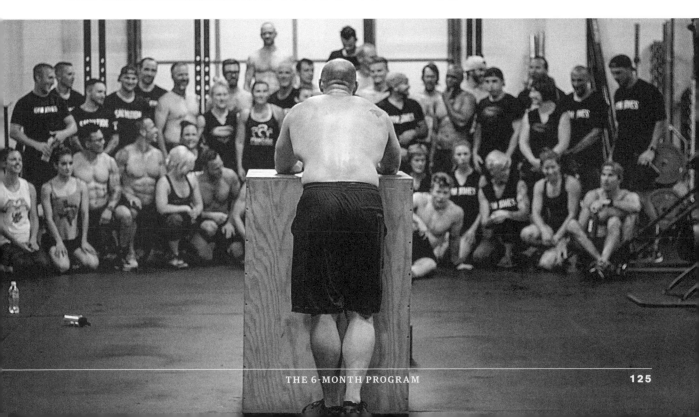

BLOCK 5

WEEKS 17 TO 20

You spent the last two blocks building strength and muscle. Now, you'll learn how to use that strength and muscle to the best of your advantage. You'll drastically improve the top end of your fitness, building an incredible ability to do a lot of devastatingly hard work in a short amount of time, a subsection of fitness called power endurance.

Monday: Warmup, Circuit-Style, Finisher, Cooldown

Tuesday: Warmup, IWT, Cooldown

Wednesday: Warmup, Interval, Finisher, Cooldown

Thursday: Warmup, IWT, Cooldown

Friday: Warmup, Circuit-Style, Finisher, Cooldown

Saturday: Rest or Warmup, Time Trial, Finisher, Cooldown

Sunday: Rest or Recovery (Cardiovascular)

BLOCK 6

WEEKS 21 TO 24

This is the final block of the program. In this block, you'll continue to improve all aspects of your fitness, and you'll fill any lingering holes. You'll also retest yourself to see just how much you've improved over nearly 6 months of hard training.

Monday: Warmup, Max Test or Challenge, Finisher, Cooldown

Tuesday: Warmup, Time Trial, Cooldown

Wednesday: Warmup, Max Test or Challenge, Finisher, Cooldown

Thursday: Warmup, Interval, Finisher, Cooldown

Friday: Warmup, Circuit-Style, Finisher, Cooldown

Saturday: Rest or Warmup, IWT, Finisher, Cooldown

Sunday: Rest or Recovery (Cardiovascular)

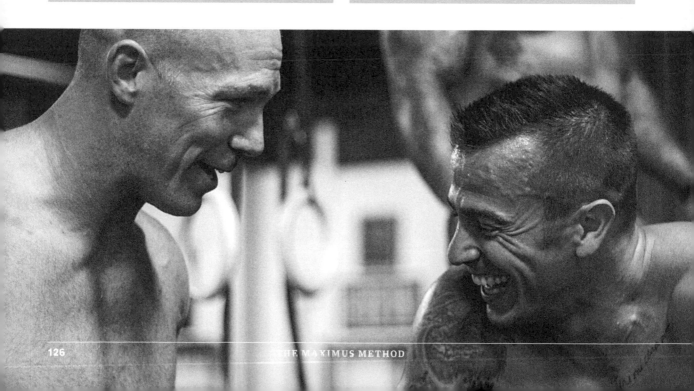

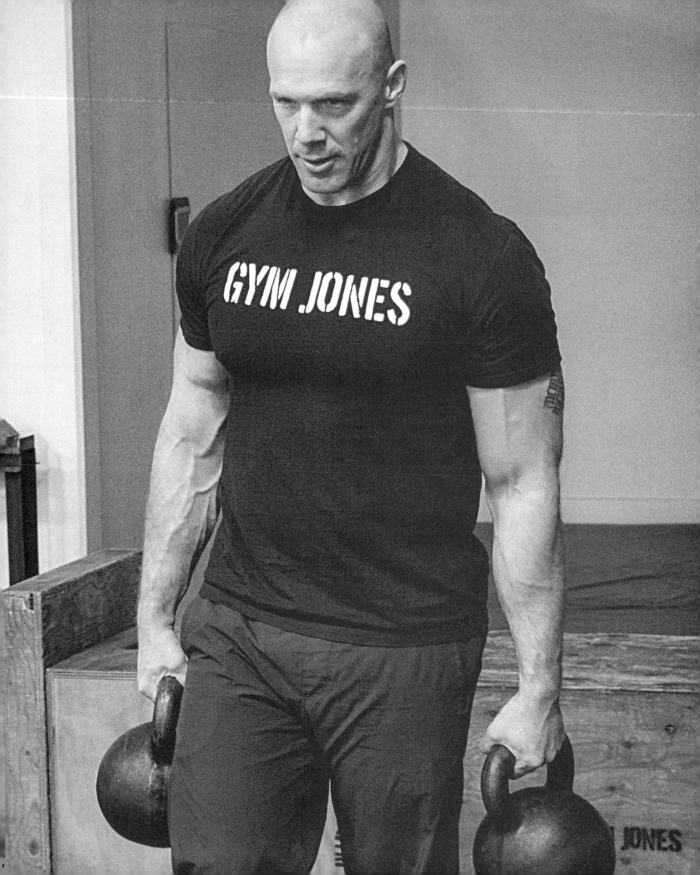

Don't quit. EVER.

THE 12-WEEK PROGRAM

This program is broken down into three blocks, each focusing on a different aspect of overall fitness.

Each week contains approximately 11 hours of training, and most of the workouts should take only an hour. You'll train 6 days a week, doing two training sessions on 5 of those days, and one on the sixth day. Each 4-week block gives you 1 week of training. So, you'll repeat that week for 4 weeks, then move on to the next block.

The first block of training—weeks 1 to 4— focuses on testing your strength, building a base level of strength and stamina, and reaching a high level of cardiovascular fitness.

The second block of training—weeks 5 to 8—is centered on helping you become stronger and trading your fat for muscle, which is necessary if you're trying to lose weight or look better.

The final block of training—weeks 9 to 12— teaches you how to use the strength and muscle you've built in the past blocks. You'll increase your cardiovascular fitness, and also move like an athlete.

When you look at this program, it may seem like a lot of work. It is. Big goals require big measures. This program takes a great deal of effort, but if you want to become incredibly fit in a short amount of time, this is what it takes.

Depending on your starting level, you may be sore, and you may become tired. My advice: Work that much harder on your recovery practices, and sleep more.

HOW IT WORKS

I've provided you with a predetermined program, including the exact warmup, workout, finisher, and cooldown that you should do on each day for the full 12 weeks. Because you're chasing a difficult goal, I don't want you to have to think about what your workout should look like. I've recommended the best training session for each day. All you have to do is show up and work hard.

Immediately following each block, I've also provided you with a template so that you can build your own training sessions if you prefer to, or need to. In the event that you can't do the workout I recommend, this allows you to make substitutions so you can still improve.

So, for example, let's say that on a Tuesday a.m. workout, I recommend that you do "Time Trial 4: Max Meters in 30," a workout that includes a rowing or skiing machine. But if you go to the gym and all the machines are taken, you'd go to the given week's template, and see that it calls for a time trial workout. Then, you'd go to Section V: The Maximus Manual (page 149) and find the "X: Time Trials" section (page 215), and pick one that you can do, such as "Time Trial 1: 1.5-mile run." The template is an excuse-killer: You'll always be able to complete a workout.

ESSENTIAL RULES

As you go through the program, these guidelines will boost your success.

1. Don't miss days.

As you know, 12 weeks isn't long. If you want this program to work, you need to be strict. If you can't make it to the gym, you must complete one of the workouts from "VI: No-Gear Workouts" on page 190.

2. Be strict with your nutrition.

In the nutrition section, I discussed how it's okay to indulge as long as you follow the Maximus 90-percent rule. That doesn't apply to this program. When you are trying to make an extreme transformation, there is no room for error. You'll need to monitor calories and make sure every meal is on point.

3. Prioritize recovery.

This training program is taxing. If you don't take action to ensure that you recover, you're only going to crash. Sleep 8 to 9 hours each night, do something that reduces your stress, and do at least two recovery practices each day.

4. Don't lose sight of your goal.

I know this program asks a lot, but that's the cost of success. Anytime you feel overwhelmed, remember the reason you took on this challenge in the first place. In fact, write it down as a concrete reminder. Remember that there are countless people who've completed this program and completely overhauled their bodies and lives. You can be one of those people.

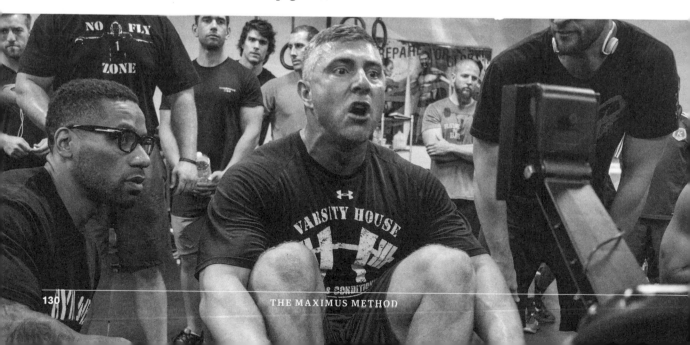

THE PROGRAM

BLOCK 1
WEEKS 1 TO 4

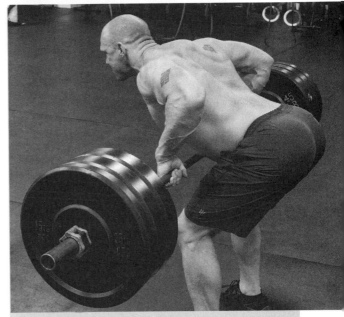

Testing and General Fitness

In this block, you'll increase your general fitness and test your limitations. I believe in testing, for a few reasons. First, as the program progresses, it's important that you use the correct weight in certain workouts, and these tests help you to determine which weights to use. (You'll need to know your 1-rep max to determine which weights to use in some workouts.) Second, you need to know where you're starting. It's incredibly motivating and interesting to look back at your old numbers and see just how far you have come. Third, and most important, testing tells you where your limits are. Once you have those, you'll know how hard you will need to work to push past them, which is exactly what you need to do to see physical and mental change.

When you do the "Max Test" workouts, make sure that you perform each of the max tests, including the barbell bench press, barbell overhead press, barbell deadlift, barbell front squat, barbell back squat, and barbell overhead squat. Once you've determined your numbers on all of the max tests, you can do challenge workouts on days that call for max tests.

WORKOUT TEMPLATE

Monday A.M.: Warmup, Max Test, Finisher, Cooldown

Monday P.M.: Recovery (Cardiovascular)

Tuesday A.M.: Warmup, Time Trial, Cooldown

Tuesday P.M.: Recovery (Cardiovascular)

Wednesday A.M.: Warmup, Max Test or Challenge, Finisher, Cooldown

Wednesday P.M.: Recovery (Cardiovascular)

Thursday A.M.: Warmup, Death By, Finisher, Cooldown

Thursday P.M.: Recovery (Cardiovascular)

Friday A.M.: Warmup, Challenge, Finisher, Cooldown

Friday P.M.: Warmup, Circuit-Style, Finisher, Cooldown

Saturday: Warmup, Interval, Cooldown

Sunday: Rest or Recovery

BLOCK 2
WEEKS 5 TO 8

Strength and Power

Block 1 increased your general fitness and gave you a solid foundation. Now it's time to build some serious horsepower. This block of training focuses on improving your strength, power, and muscle mass while maintaining your cardiovascular fitness. I've structured the workouts so that your muscle groups can recover as much as possible in between sessions, so your body is ready to go hard every workout. By the end of this block, you'll look better and feel capable of anything.

WORKOUT TEMPLATE

Monday A.M.: Warmup, Strength and Power, Finisher, Cooldown

Monday P.M.: Recovery (Cardiovascular)

Tuesday A.M.: Warmup, Mass Gain, Finisher, Cooldown

Tuesday P.M.: Warmup, Interval, Cooldown

Wednesday A.M.: Warmup, Strength and Power, Finisher, Cooldown

Wednesday P.M.: Recovery (Cardiovascular)

Thursday A.M.: Warmup, Mass Gain, Finisher, Cooldown

Thursday P.M.: Warmup, Time Trial, Cooldown

Friday A.M.: Warmup, Circuit-Style, Finisher, Cooldown

Friday P.M.: Warmup, Interval, Cooldown

Saturday: Warmup, IWT, Cooldown

Sunday: Rest or Recovery

BLOCK 3
WEEKS 9 TO 12

Cardiovascular Fitness

You're almost there. In Block 3, you'll build incredible fitness, learn to move like an athlete, and forge a high level of endurance and work capacity. This block is where your fitness really starts to blossom. By the end of this phase, you'll be tired, but you'll feel better than you ever have and ready for whatever comes next. There is a lot of breathing work in this block, and the key is to push yourself as hard as humanly possible workout after workout.

WORKOUT TEMPLATE

Monday A.M.: Warmup, Strength and Power, Finisher, Cooldown

Monday P.M.: Warmup, Interval, Cooldown

Tuesday A.M.: Warmup, Circuit-Style, Finisher, Cooldown

Tuesday P.M.: Recovery (Cardiovascular)

Wednesday A.M.: Warmup, IWT, Cooldown

Wednesday P.M.: Warmup, Time Trial, Cooldown

Thursday A.M.: Warmup, Interval, Cooldown

Thursday P.M.: Recovery (Weighted)

Friday A.M.: Warmup, Circuit-Style, Finisher, Cooldown

Friday P.M.: Warmup, IWT, Cooldown

Saturday: Warmup, Challenge, Finisher, Cooldown

Sunday: Rest or Recovery

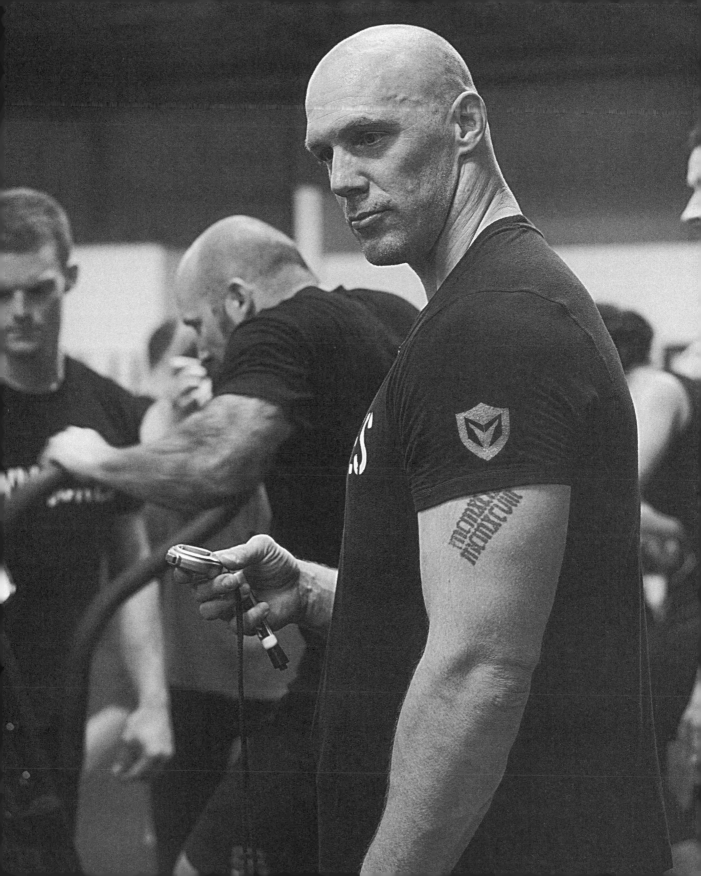

BLOCK 1: WEEKS 1–2

WEEK 1

MONDAY A.M.
Warmup 1: LBD (page 154)
Max Test 3: Barbell Deadlift (page 159)
Finisher 6: Pullup Ladder (page 222)
Cooldown (page 233)

MONDAY P.M.
Recovery 3: Fartlek Fun (page 230)

TUESDAY A.M.
Warmup 3: Interval Warmup (page 155)
Time Trial 2: 5K Run (page 215)
Cooldown (page 233)

TUESDAY P.M.
Recovery 2: Easy Intervals (page 228)

WEDNESDAY A.M.
Warmup 2: Total Body (page 154)
Max Test 4: Barbell Front Squat (page 159)
Finisher 2: 1K Row (page 220)
Cooldown (page 233)

WEDNESDAY P.M.
Recovery 1: 60 at 70 (page 228)

THURSDAY A.M.
Warmup 6: Quick Warmup (page 156)
Death by 1: Death by Burpee (page 175)
Finisher 9: 50QR (page 225)
Cooldown (page 233)

THURSDAY P.M.
Recovery 3: Fartlek Fun (page 230)

FRIDAY A.M.
Warmup 3: Interval Warmup (page 155)
Challenge 1: 2K Row (page 205)
Finisher 7: 5-Minute Plank (page 224)
Cooldown (page 233)

FRIDAY P.M.
Warmup 1: LBD (page 154)
Circuit-Style 10: Don't Ask Me about Your Abs (page 166)
Finisher 10: The Best for Last (page 225)
Cooldown (page 233)

SATURDAY
Warmup 3: Interval Warmup (page 155)
Interval 1: 30/30 (page 179)
Cooldown (page 233)

SUNDAY
Rest or Recovery

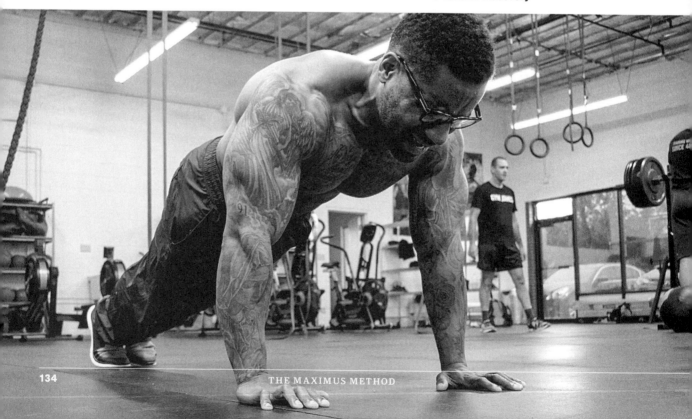

WEEK 2

MONDAY A.M.
Warmup 4: UBD (page 155)
Max Test 1: Barbell Bench Press (page 159)
Finisher 1: 500-Meter Row (page 220)
Cooldown (page 233)

MONDAY P.M.
Recovery 1: 60 at 70 (page 228)

TUESDAY A.M.
Warmup 3: Interval Warmup (page 155)
Time Trial 1: 1.5-Mile Run (page 215)
Cooldown (page 233)

TUESDAY P.M.
Recovery 3: Fartlek Fun (page 230)

WEDNESDAY A.M.
Warmup 4: UBD (page 155)
Max Test 2: Barbell Overhead Press (page 159)
Finisher 4: 1-Miler (page 221)
Cooldown (page 233)

WEDNESDAY P.M.
Recovery 2: Easy Intervals (page 228)

THURSDAY A.M.
Warmup 7: Maximus Warmup (page 157)
Death by 4: Death by Air Squat (page 176)
Finisher 5: Quick and Dirty (page 222)
Cooldown (page 233)

THURSDAY P.M.
Recovery 1: 60 at 70 (page 228)

FRIDAY A.M.
Warmup 4: UBD (page 155)
Challenge 2: 100 Burpees for Time (page 205)
Finisher 1: 500-Meter Row (page 220)
Cooldown (page 233)

FRIDAY P.M.
Warmup 5: Olympic Warmup (page 156)
Circuit-Style 11: EDIMFSD (page 167)
Finisher 7: 5-Minute Plank (page 224)
Cooldown (page 233)

SATURDAY
Warmup 3: Interval Warmup (page 155)
Interval 2: 500-Meter Murder (page 179)
Cooldown (page 233)

SUNDAY
Rest or Recovery

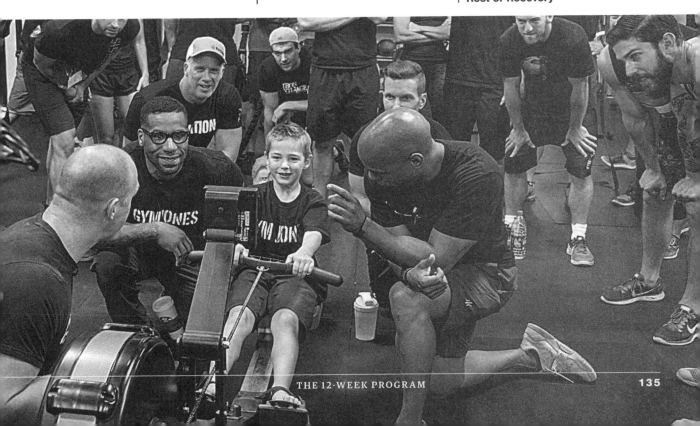

BLOCK 1: WEEKS 3-4

WEEK 3

MONDAY A.M.
Warmup 1: LBD (page 154)
Max Test 5: Barbell Back Squat (page 159)
Finisher 3: 300FY (page 221)
Cooldown (page 233)

MONDAY P.M.
Recovery 2: Easy Intervals (page 228)

TUESDAY A.M.
Warmup 3: Interval Warmup (page 155)
Time Trial 4: Max Meters in 30 (page 216)
Cooldown (page 233)

TUESDAY P.M.
Recovery 3: Fartlek Fun (page 230)

WEDNESDAY A.M.
Warmup 3: Interval Warmup (page 155)
Challenge 1: 2K Row (page 205)
Finisher 7: 5-Minute Plank (page 224)
Cooldown (page 233)

WEDNESDAY P.M.
Recovery 1: 60 at 70 (page 228)

THURSDAY A.M.
Warmup 4: UBD (page 155)
Death by 3: Death by Pushup (page 176)
Finisher 5: Quick and Dirty (page 222)
Cooldown (page 233)

THURSDAY P.M.
Recovery 3: Fartlek Fun (page 230)

FRIDAY A.M.
Warmup 2: Total Body (page 154)
Challenge 6: The Treadmill Drill (page 207)
Finisher 7: 5-Minute Plank (page 224)
Cooldown (page 233)

FRIDAY P.M.
Warmup 1: LBD (page 154)
Circuit-Style 6: Gut Punch (page 164)
Finisher 1: 500-Meter Row (page 220)
Cooldown (page 233)

SATURDAY
Warmup 3: Interval Warmup (page 155)
Interval 4: Row to Hell (page 180)
Cooldown (page 233)

SUNDAY
Rest or Recovery

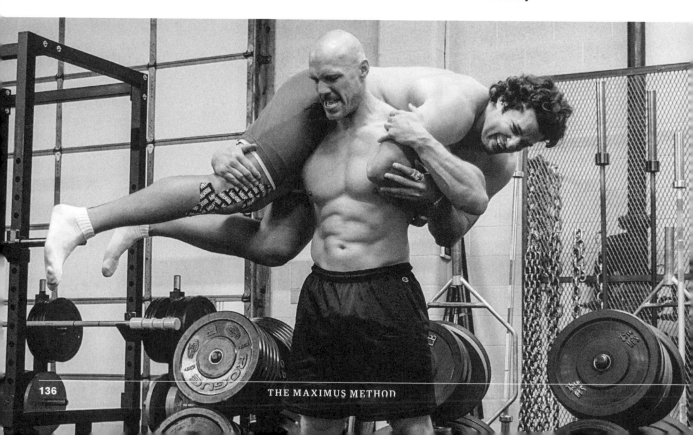

WEEK 4

MONDAY A.M.
Warmup 2: Total Body (page 154)
Max Test 6: Barbell Overhead Squat (page 159)
Finisher 5: Quick and Dirty (page 222)
Cooldown (page 233)

MONDAY P.M.
Recovery 2: Easy Intervals (page 228)

TUESDAY A.M.
Warmup 3: Interval Warmup (page 155)
Time Trial 5: Max Meters In 60 (page 217)
Cooldown (page 233)

TUESDAY P.M.
Recovery 3: Fartlek Fun (page 230)

WEDNESDAY A.M.
Warmup 7: Maximus Warmup (page 157)
Challenge 3: Can't vs. Won't (page 206)
Finisher 9: 50QR (page 225)
Cooldown (page 233)

WEDNESDAY P.M.
Recovery 1: 60 at 70 (page 228)

THURSDAY A.M.
Warmup 2: Total Body (page 154)
Death by 4: Death by Air Squat (page 176)
Finisher 2: 1K Row (page 220)
Cooldown (page 233)

THURSDAY P.M.
Recovery 2: Easy Intervals (page 228)

FRIDAY A.M.
Warmup 7: Maximus Warmup (page 157)
Challenge 14: Sacrament (page 211)
Finisher 3: 300FY (page 221)
Cooldown (page 233)

FRIDAY P.M.
Warmup 4: UBD (page 155)
Circuit-Style 5: Welcome Party (page 164)
Finisher 9: 50QR (page 225)
Cooldown (page 233)

SATURDAY
Warmup 3: Interval Warmup (page 155)
Interval 7: Add a Meter (page 182)
Cooldown (page 233)

SUNDAY
Rest or Recovery

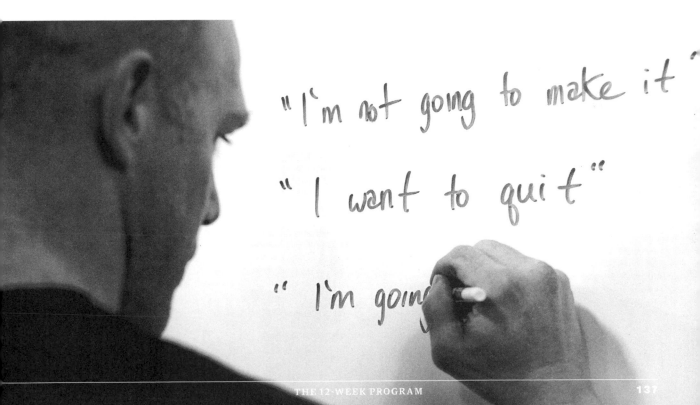

"I'm not going to make it"

"I want to quit"

"I'm going

BLOCK 2: WEEKS 5-6

WEEK 5

MONDAY A.M.
Warmup 1: LBD (page 154)
Strength and Power 1: 5 by 2 at 80–Barbell Front Squat (page 200)
Finisher 1: 500-Meter Row (page 220)
Cooldown (page 233)

MONDAY P.M.
Recovery 2: Easy Intervals (page 228)

TUESDAY A.M.
Warmup 4: UBD (page 155)
Mass Gain 1: 10 by 10 Upper (page 188)
Finisher 2: 1K Row (page 220)
Cooldown (page 233)

TUESDAY P.M.
Warmup 3: Interval Warmup (page 155)
Interval 8: Wheels (page 182)
Cooldown (page 233)

WEDNESDAY A.M.
Warmup 6: Quick Warmup (page 156)
Strength and Power 1: 5 by 2 at 80–Barbell Back Squat (page 200)
Finisher 7: 5-Minute Plank (page 224)
Cooldown (page 233)

WEDNESDAY P.M.
Recovery 3: Fartlek Fun (page 230)

THURSDAY A.M.
Warmup 4: UBD (page 155)
Mass Gain 4: Ticket to Gainzville (page 189)
Finisher 4: 1-Miler (page 221)
Cooldown (page 233)

THURSDAY P.M.
Warmup 3: Interval Warmup (page 155)
Time Trial 5: Max Meters in 60 (page 217)
Cooldown (page 233)

FRIDAY A.M.
Warmup 5: Olympic Warmup (page 156)
Circuit-Style 15: Load and Explode (page 169)
Finisher 10: The Best for Last (page 225)
Cooldown (page 233)

FRIDAY P.M.
Warmup 3: Interval Warmup (page 155)
Interval 3: Fan Bike to Hell (page 180)
Cooldown (page 233)

SATURDAY
Warmup 2: Total Body (page 154)
IWT 2: Strength (page 186)
Cooldown (page 233)

SUNDAY
Rest or Recovery

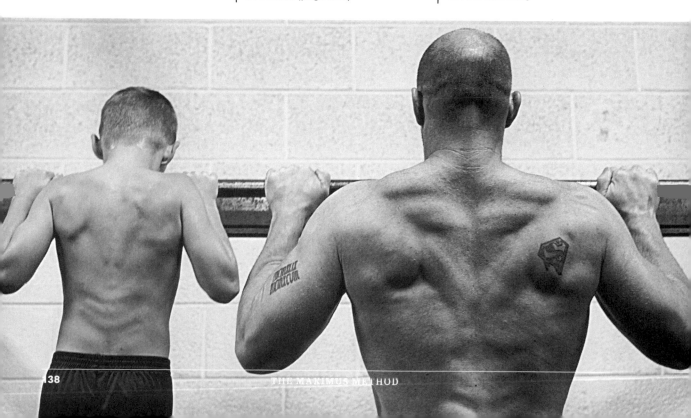

WEEK 6

MONDAY A.M.
Warmup 4: UBD (page 155)
Strength and Power 5: Add 5 (page 202)
Finisher 9: 50QR (page 225)
Cooldown (page 233)

MONDAY P.M.
Recovery 1: 60 at 70 (page 228)

TUESDAY A.M.
Warmup 1: LBD (page 154)
Mass Gain 2: 10 by 10 Lower (page 188)
Finisher 5: Quick and Dirty (page 222)
Cooldown (page 233)

TUESDAY P.M.
Warmup 3: Interval Warmup (page 155)
Interval 9: Tabata Triplets (page 183)
Cooldown (page 233)

WEDNESDAY A.M.
Warmup 4: UBD (page 155)
Strength and Power 2: 6 by 2 at 85–Barbell Bench Press (page 200)
Finisher 8: Pushup Maximus (page 224)
Cooldown (page 233)

WEDNESDAY P.M.
Recovery 3: Fartlek Fun (page 230)

THURSDAY A.M.
Warmup 6: Quick Warmup (page 156)
Mass Gain 3: 4 by 15–Barbell Front Squat (page 189)
Finisher 2: 1K Row (page 220)
Cooldown (page 233)

THURSDAY P.M.
Warmup 3: Interval Warmup (page 155)
Time Trial 1: 1.5-Mile Run (page 215)
Cooldown (page 233)

FRIDAY A.M.
Warmup 4: UBD (page 155)
Circuit-Style 1: The Holy Trinity (page 162)
Finisher 1: 500-Meter Row (page 220)
Cooldown (page 233)

FRIDAY P.M.
Warmup 3: Interval Warmup (page 155)
Interval 5: Let's Make a Deal (page 181)
Cooldown (page 233)

SATURDAY
Warmup 7: Maximus Warmup (page 157)
IWT 1: General (page 186)
Cooldown (page 233)

SUNDAY
Rest or Recovery

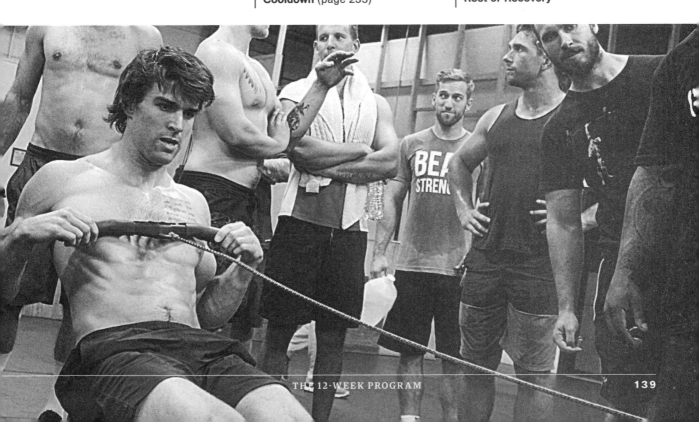

BLOCK 2: WEEKS 7-8

WEEK 7

MONDAY A.M.
Warmup 1: LBD (page 154)
Strength and Power 1: 5 by 2 at 80–Barbell Back Squat (page 200)
Finisher 7: 5-Minute Plank (page 224)
Cooldown (page 233)

MONDAY P.M.
Recovery 2: Easy Intervals (page 228)

TUESDAY A.M.
Warmup 4: UBD (page 155)
Mass Gain 3: 4 by 15–Barbell Bench Press (page 189)
Finisher 6: Pullup Ladder (page 222)
Cooldown (page 233)

TUESDAY P.M.
Warmup 3: Interval Warmup (page 155)
Interval 10: Time Bomb (page 183)
Cooldown (page 233)

WEDNESDAY A.M.
Warmup 5: Olympic Warmup (page 156)
Strength and Power 9: Rocket Boosters (page 204)
Finisher 1: 500-Meter Row (page 220)
Cooldown (page 233)

WEDNESDAY P.M.
Recovery 1: 60 at 70 (page 228)

THURSDAY A.M.
Warmup 4: UBD (page 155)
Mass Gain 1: 10 by 10 Upper (page 188)
Finisher 5: Quick and Dirty (page 222)
Cooldown (page 233)

THURSDAY P.M.
Warmup 3: Interval Warmup (page 155)
Time Trial 2: 5K Run (page 215)
Cooldown (page 233)

FRIDAY A.M.
Warmup 6: Quick Warmup (page 156)
Circuit-Style 18: It's Tricky (page 170)
Finisher 7: 5-Minute Plank (page 224)
Cooldown (page 233)

FRIDAY P.M.
Warmup 3: Interval Warmup (page 155)
Interval 6: The Long Road (page 181)
Cooldown (page 233)

SATURDAY
Warmup 5: Olympic Warmup (page 156)
IWT 3: Endurance (page 187)
Cooldown (page 233)

SUNDAY
Rest or Recovery

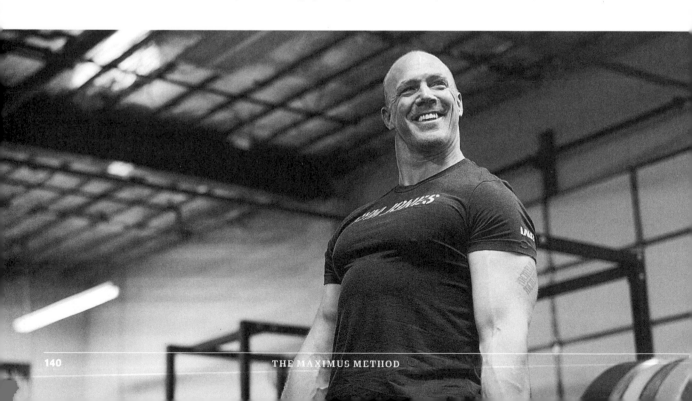

WEEK 8

MONDAY A.M.
Warmup 4: UBD (page 155)
Strength and Power 6: 100-Rep Challenge–Barbell Bench Press (page 202)
Finisher 2: 1K Row (page 220)
Cooldown (page 233)

MONDAY P.M.
Recovery 3: Fartlek Fun (page 230)

TUESDAY A.M.
Warmup 1: LBD (page 154)
Mass Gain 3: 4 by 15–Barbell Front Squat (page 189)
Finisher 3: 300FY (page 221)
Cooldown (page 233)

TUESDAY P.M.
Warmup 3: Interval Warmup (page 155)
Interval 11: Fight Test (page 184)
Cooldown (page 233)

WEDNESDAY A.M.
Warmup 4: UBD (page 155)
Strength and Power 3: 4 by 4 at 80–Barbell Overhead Press (page 201)
Finisher 8: Pushup Maximus (page 224)
Cooldown (page 233)

WEDNESDAY P.M.
Recovery 1: 60 at 70 (page 228)

THURSDAY A.M.
Warmup 6: Quick Warmup (page 156)
Mass Gain 2: 10 by 10 Lower (page 188)
Finisher 7: 5-Minute Plank (page 224)
Cooldown (page 233)

THURSDAY P.M.
Warmup 3: Interval Warmup (page 155)
Time Trial 3: Make Weight (page 216)
Cooldown (page 233)

FRIDAY A.M.
Warmup 4: UBD (page 155)
Circuit-Style 2: Love/Hate (page 162)
Finisher 10: The Best for Last (page 225)
Cooldown (page 233)

FRIDAY P.M.
Warmup 3: Interval Warmup (page 155)
Interval 2: 500-Meter Murder (page 179)
Cooldown (page 233)

SATURDAY
Warmup 7: Maximus Warmup (page 157)
IWT 2: Strength (page 186)
Cooldown (page 233)

SUNDAY
Rest or Recovery

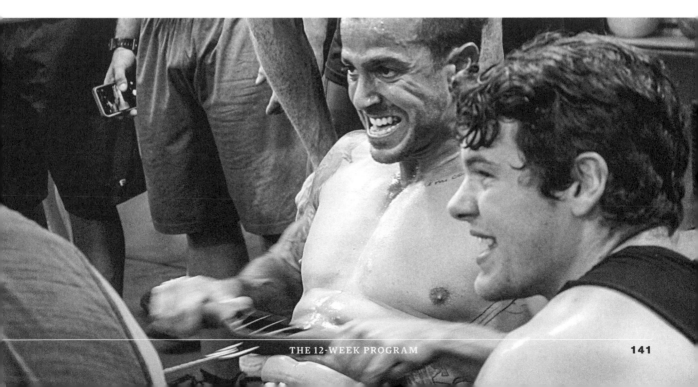

BLOCK 3: WEEKS 9-10

WEEK 9

MONDAY A.M.
Warmup 1: LBD (page 154)
Strength and Power 1: 5 by 2 at 80–Barbell Deadlift (page 200)
Finisher 1: 500-Meter Row (page 220)
Cooldown (page 233)

MONDAY P.M.
Warmup 3: Interval Warmup (page 155)
Interval 1: 30/30 (page 179)
Cooldown (page 233)

TUESDAY A.M.
Warmup 4: UBD (page 155)
Circuit-Style 1: The Holy Trinity (page 162)
Finisher 2: 1K Row (page 220)
Cooldown (page 233)

TUESDAY P.M.
Recovery 1: 60 at 70 (page 228)

WEDNESDAY A.M.
Warmup 5: Olympic Warmup (page 156)
IWT 2: Strength (page 186)
Cooldown (page 233)

WEDNESDAY P.M.
Warmup 3: Interval Warmup (page 155)
Time Trial 2: 5K Run (page 215)
Cooldown (page 233)

THURSDAY A.M.
Warmup 3: Interval Warmup (page 155)
Interval 2: 500-Meter Murder (page 179)
Cooldown (page 233)

THURSDAY P.M.
Recovery 4: Upper-Body Recovery (page 230)

FRIDAY A.M.
Warmup 6: Quick Warmup (page 156)
Circuit-Style 3: 400-Meter Manslaughter (page 163)
Finisher 7: 5-Minute Plank (page 224)
Cooldown (page 233)

FRIDAY P.M.
Warmup 7: Maximus Warmup (page 157)
IWT 1: General (page 186)
Cooldown (page 233)

SATURDAY
Warmup 3: Interval Warmup (page 155)
Challenge 3: Can't vs. Won't (page 206)
Finisher 8: Pushup Maximus (page 224)
Cooldown (page 233)

SUNDAY
Rest or Recovery

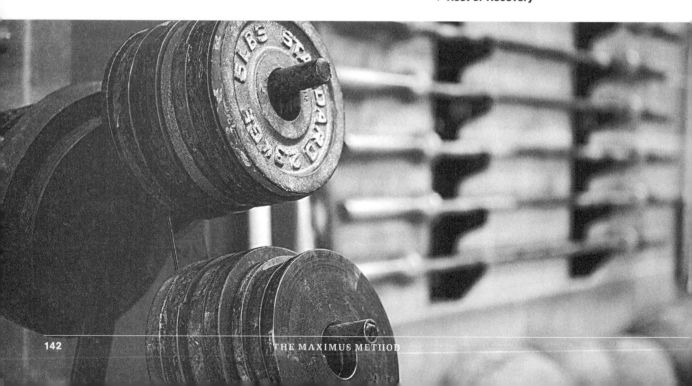

WEEK 10

MONDAY A.M.
Warmup 5: Olympic Warmup (page 156)
Strength and Power 7: Speed Kills (page 203)
Finisher 1: 500-Meter Row (page 220)
Cooldown (page 233)

MONDAY P.M.
Warmup 3: Interval Warmup (page 155)
Interval 4: Row to Hell (page 180)
Cooldown (page 233)

TUESDAY A.M.
Warmup 2: Total Body (page 154)
Circuit-Style 7: Circus Maximus (page 165)
Finisher 2: 1K Row (page 220)
Cooldown (page 233)

TUESDAY P.M.
Recovery 3: Fartlek Fun (page 230)

WEDNESDAY A.M.
Warmup 7: Maximus Warmup (page 157)
IWT 3: Endurance (page 187)
Cooldown (page 233)

WEDNESDAY P.M.
Warmup 3: Interval Warmup (page 155)
Time Trial 5: Max Meters in 60 (page 217)
Cooldown (page 233)

THURSDAY A.M.
Warmup 3: Interval Warmup (page 155)
Interval 5: Let's Make a Deal (page 181)
Cooldown (page 233)

THURSDAY P.M.
Recovery 5: 100 Turkish Getups (page 231)

FRIDAY A.M.
Warmup 2: Total Body (page 154)
Circuit-Style 4: Five-Fifty Five (page 163)
Finisher 7: 5-Minute Plank (page 224)
Cooldown (page 233)

FRIDAY P.M.
Warmup 6: Quick Warmup (page 156)
IWT 1: General (page 186)
Cooldown (page 233)

SATURDAY
Warmup 7: Maximus Warmup (page 157)
Challenge 18: 100 Burpee Pullups (page 213)
Finisher 9: 50QR (page 225)
Cooldown (page 233)

SUNDAY
Rest or Recovery

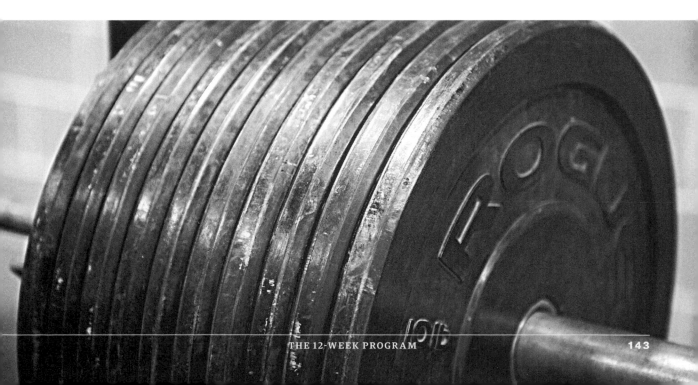

BLOCK 3: WEEKS 11-12

WEEK 11

MONDAY A.M.
Warmup 5: Olympic Warmup (page 156)
Strength and Power 2: 6 by 2 at 85–Barbell Deadlift (page 200)
Finisher 6: Pullup Ladder (page 222)
Cooldown (page 233)

MONDAY P.M.
Warmup 3: Interval Warmup (page 155)
Interval 6: The Long Road (page 181)
Cooldown (page 233)

TUESDAY A.M.
Warmup 7: Maximus Warmup (page 157)
Circuit-Style 12: Balls to the Walls (page 167)
Finisher 7: 5-Minute Plank (page 224)
Cooldown (page 233)

TUESDAY P.M.
Recovery 2: Easy Intervals (page 228)

WEDNESDAY A.M.
Warmup 2: Total Body (page 154)
IWT 1: General (page 186)
Cooldown (page 233)

WEDNESDAY P.M.
Warmup 3: Interval Warmup (page 155)
Time Trial 3: Make Weight (page 216)
Cooldown (page 233)

THURSDAY A.M.
Warmup 3: Interval Warmup (page 155)
Interval 7: Add a Meter (page 182)
Cooldown (page 233)

THURSDAY P.M.
Recovery 5: 100 Turkish Getups (page 231)

FRIDAY A.M.
Warmup 7: Maximus Warmup (page 157)
Circuit-Style 9: Opposites Attract (page 166)
Finisher 7: 5-Minute Plank (page 224)
Cooldown (page 233)

FRIDAY P.M.
Warmup 6: Quick Warmup (page 156)
IWT 3: Endurance (page 187)
Cooldown (page 233)

SATURDAY:
Warmup 1: LBD (page 154)
Challenge 19: 1-Mile Lunge (page 214)
Finisher 8: Pushup Maximus (page 224)
Cooldown (page 233)

SUNDAY:
Rest or Recovery

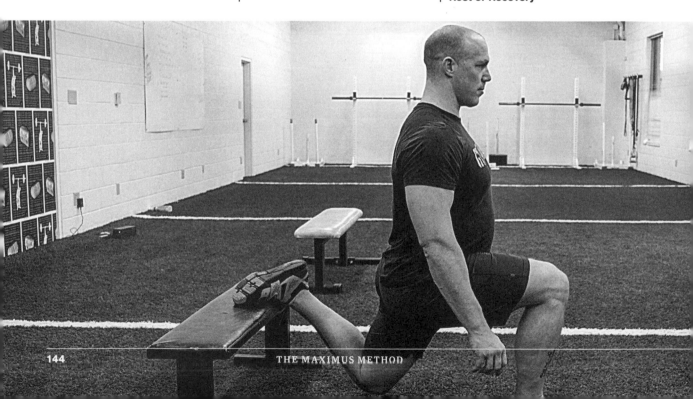

WEEK 12

MONDAY A.M.
Warmup 1: LBD (page 154)
Strength and Power 7: Speed Kills (page 203)
Finisher 1: 500-Meter Row (page 220)
Cooldown (page 233)

MONDAY P.M.
Warmup 3: Interval Warmup (page 155)
Interval 10: Time Bomb (page 183)
Cooldown (page 233)

TUESDAY A.M.
Warmup 4: UBD (page 155)
Circuit-Style 1: The Holy Trinity (page 162)
Finisher 7: 5-Minute Plank (page 224)
Cooldown (page 233)

TUESDAY P.M.
Recovery 1: 60 at 70 (page 228)

WEDNESDAY A.M.
Warmup 5: Olympic Warmup (page 156)
IWT 2: Strength (page 186)
Cooldown (page 233)

WEDNESDAY P.M.
Warmup 3: Interval Warmup (page 155)
Time Trial 4: Max Meters in 30 (page 216)
Cooldown (page 233)

THURSDAY A.M.
Warmup 3: Interval Warmup (page 155)
Interval 8: Wheels (page 182)
Cooldown (page 233)

THURSDAY P.M.
Recovery 6: Fix Your Form (page 231)

FRIDAY A.M.
Warmup 7: Maximus Warmup (page 157)
Circuit-Style 16: The Best for Last Burpee (page 169)
Finisher 7: 5-Minute Plank (page 224)
Cooldown (page 233)

FRIDAY P.M.
Warmup 2: Total Body (page 154)
IWT 1: General (page 186)
Cooldown (page 233)

SATURDAY
Warmup 3: Interval Warmup (page 155)
Challenge 1: 2K Row (page 205)
Finisher 9: 50QR (page 225)
Cooldown (page 233)

SUNDAY
Rest or Recovery

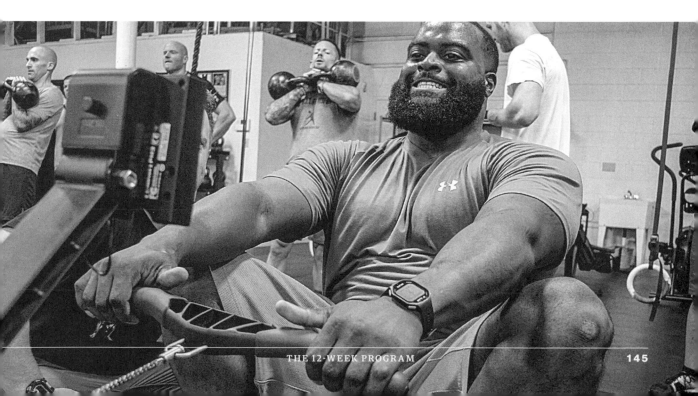

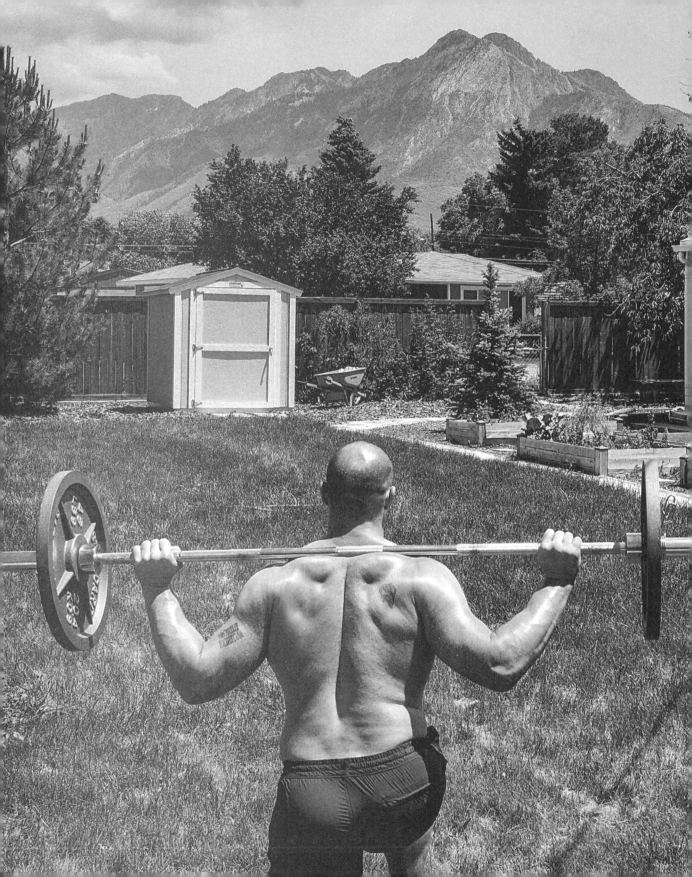

21

WEEK 25 AND BEYOND: WHAT NOW?

Whether you completed the 6-month or the 12-week program. The question inevitably becomes: What now?

You have some options, but the only option you don't have, quite frankly, is to stop training and go back to the way you were. Your journey has only just begun.

If you have finished the 6-month program, you could decide to:

A. Do it again.

B. Make a bigger commitment and do the 12-week program.

C. Decide to train every day on your own by creating your own plan and trying out all the workouts in Section V: The Maximus Manual on page 149.

If you finished the 12-week program, you could:

A. Do it again.

B. Transition into the 6-month program.

C. Decide to train every day on your own by creating your own plan and trying out all the workouts in Section V: The Maximus Manual on page 149.

Whatever you choose, don't stop. Even though you may be the most fit you've ever been in your life, you can still improve.

You have everything you need in this book to help you do just that—you have the knowledge, which is the greatest tool you could ever have. Use it.

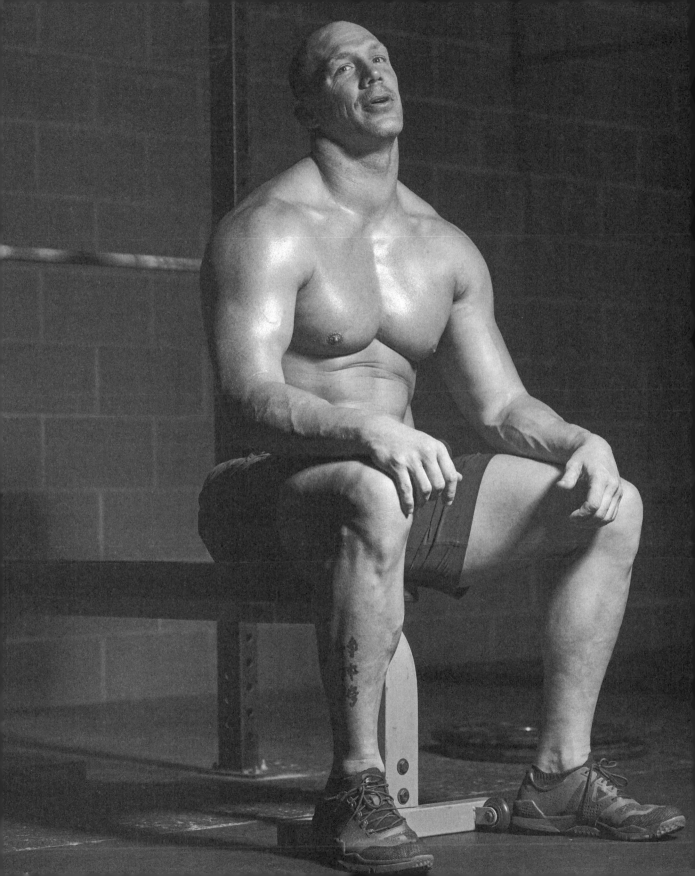

V

THE
MAXIMUS
MANUAL

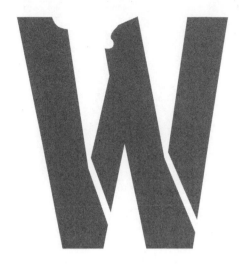

With this section, you have direct access to my brain and the knowledge I have accumulated in my years as a professional athlete and trainer.

This manual contains 100 of my favorite workouts of all time, and they're some of the most effective. I've learned a few from others, but most of them are my own.

In addition to the workouts, I've also included the world's best warmups, tests, finishers, and everything else you will need to design a full training plan that will completely overhaul your body and mind.

Let's get to work.

Bobby's Law:
Pain leads to power.
Struggle leads to strength.

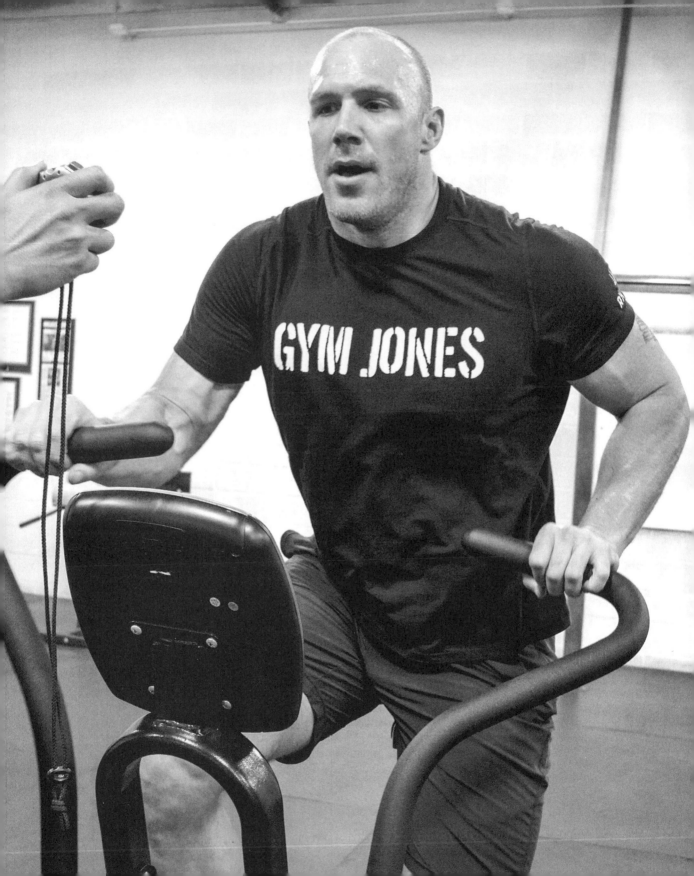

22

WARMUPS

Warmups are essential. You can't just go from sitting to an all-out effort, unless your goal is to hurt yourself. Sometimes, when I explain this at seminars, someone responds by saying, "Well, lions do that all the time." My response? "You're not a fucking lion."

Besides helping you to prevent injury, a good warmup can also make your workout more productive. A warm, loose body performs better.

There are two basic types of warmups: general and specific.

A general warmup is typically a short, easy cardio effort that signals to your body that it's time to start moving and working. You can do it on any cardio machine, or you can just run or do some basic body-weight movements.

A specific warmup prepares you for the specific training session that you're doing that day. If you're doing intervals, for example, you might do some short sprints. If you're doing upper-body lifts like the bench press, you might do some light upper-body exercises, honing your technique.

In this part, you'll find a few specific warmups that I regularly do at the gym. You'll learn how to pair them with workouts included in this book. Each includes a 10-minute cardiovascular general warmup, which you do at a low intensity. If you don't have time, you can cut the general warmup, but don't make it a habit. It's important.

Warmup 1
LBD

Do this LBD—short for lower-body day—warmup before any lower-body lifting or jump-intensive workout. It'll wake up and mobilize your hips and legs, helping you to produce more strength and power and avoid injury.

DIRECTIONS

Start with an easy general warmup. Then, do all the sets and reps of the exercises in the order shown. Rest for 10 to 20 seconds between sets, or as needed.

1. Easy-Pace Row, Run, Bike, Stair-Climb: 10 Minutes

2. Wall Squat: 3 Sets, 5 Reps

3. Air Squat: 3 Sets, 20 Reps

4. Goblet Squat: 3 Sets, 5 Reps

5. Body-Weight Lunge: 3 Sets, 20 Meters

6. Dumbbell Overhead Lunge: 3 Sets, 20 Meters (10-Pound Dumbbells)

7. Jump Squat: 5 Sets, 5 Reps

Time: 20 Minutes

Warmup 2
TOTAL BODY

This warmup activates and loosens every single muscle in your body and has you move in every direction. I do it before any weighted workout where I'll be working my entire body.

DIRECTIONS

Start with an easy general warmup. Then, do all your sets and reps of exercises 2, 3, and 4 in the order shown. Rest for 10 to 20 seconds between sets, or as needed. Next, do the barbell complex as a circuit: without ever setting the barbell down, do 6 reps of exercise 5A, 6 reps of exercise 5B, 6 reps of exercise 5C, and so on, all the way down to exercise 5F. That's one set. Do a total of 3 sets, using slightly heavier weight each set.

1. Easy-Pace Row, Run, Bike, Stair-Climb: 10 Minutes

2. Wall Squat: 3 Sets, 5 Reps

3. Air Squat: 3 Sets, 20 Reps

4. Goblet Squat: 3 Sets, 5 Reps

5A. Barbell Deadlift: 3 Sets, 6 Reps

5B. Barbell Bent Row: 3 Sets, 6 Reps

5C. Barbell Hang Clean: 3 Sets, 6 Reps

5D. Barbell Front Squat: 3 Sets, 6 Reps

5E. Barbell Push Press: 3 Sets, 6 Reps

5F. Barbell Back Squat: 3 Sets, 6 Reps

Time: 20 Minutes

Warmup 3
INTERVAL WARMUP

This will prep your body for any high-intensity interval workout, allowing you to go faster, longer.

DIRECTIONS

Start with an easy general warmup. Then run, row, stair-climb, or bike for 30 seconds. Rest for 30 seconds. That's one round. Do 6.

1. Easy-Pace Row, Run, Bike, Stair-Climb: 10 Minutes
2A. Run, Row, Stair-Climb, Bike: 30 Seconds (6 Rounds)
2B. Rest: 30 Seconds (6 Rounds)

Time: 20 Minutes

Warmup 4
UBD

Do this UBD—short for upper-body day—warmup before any workout that's heavy on upper-body lifts. It, for example, is perfect for any bench press or pull-up test.

DIRECTIONS

Start with a general warmup, then do all the sets and reps of the exercises in the order shown.

For exercises 3A and 3B, do each exercise for 30 seconds: 30 seconds of push presses and 30 seconds of overhead holds is one round. Two rounds is one "block." Do 3 blocks, resting for 1 minute between blocks, then continue through the list.

1. Easy-Pace Row, Run, Bike, Stair-Climb: 10 Minutes
2. Shoulder Dislocate: 3 Sets, 10 Reps
3A. Dumbbell Push Press: 30 Seconds (3 Blocks, 2 Rounds Each) — **(3 Blocks)**
3B. Dumbbell Overhead Hold: 30 Seconds (3 Blocks, 2 Rounds Each)
4. Pushup: 3 Sets, 10 Reps
5. Pullup: 5 Sets, 5 Reps

Time: 20 Minutes

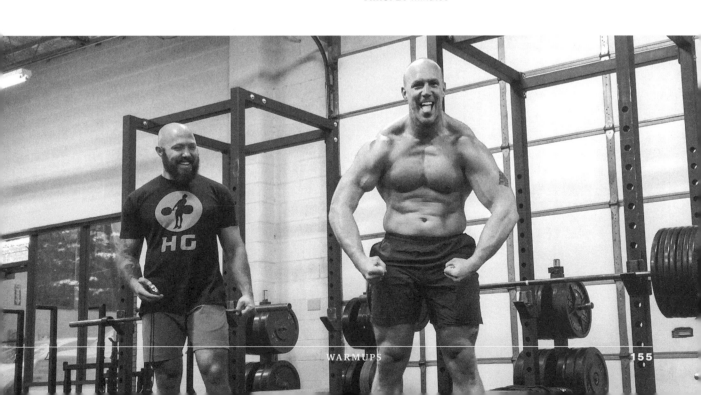

Warmup 5
OLYMPIC WARMUP

In this warmup, use a light barbell to practice a few explosive lifts. It not only readies your muscles for work but it also improves your technique, allowing you to use better form in your warmup. Use it for any workout that includes explosive lifts.

DIRECTIONS

Start with a general warmup. Load a barbell so it weighs 75 pounds. Do 1 clean, 1 front squat, and 1 hang clean. That's 1 round. Complete 1 round every 30 seconds for 10 minutes.

1. Easy-Pace Row, Run, Bike, Stair-Climb: 10 Minutes
2A. Barbell Clean: 1 Rep Every 30 Seconds
2B. Barbell Front Squat: 1 Rep Every 30 Seconds
2C. Barbell Hang Clean: 1 Rep Every 30 Seconds

Time: 20 Minutes

Warmup 6
QUICK WARMUP

Pressed for time? Do this warmup before any workout where you're just trying to get in the gym, do some quality work, and then get out. It checks off a lot of fitness boxes and readies your body in just 5 to 15 minutes.

DIRECTIONS

Start with a general warmup (if time allows). Next, do exercise 2A for 30 seconds, rest for 15 seconds (if needed); do exercise 2B for 30 seconds, and rest for 15 seconds; do exercise 2C for 30 seconds, rest for 15 seconds, and so on, all the way down to exercise 2G. That's 1 round. Do 1 to 2 rounds.

1. Easy-Pace Row, Run, Bike, Stair-Climb: 5 Minutes
2A. Air Squat: 30 Seconds
2B. Jump Squat: 30 Seconds
2C. Wall Sit: 30 Seconds
2D. Lunge: 30 Seconds
2E. Frog Hop: 30 Seconds
2F. Split Jump: 30 Seconds
2G. Burpee: 30 Seconds

Time: 5 to 15 Minutes

Warmup 7
MAXIMUS WARMUP

This should be your go-to warmup. It requires just two light dumbbells (15 to 25 pounds each), but preps your entire body for any hard workout.

DIRECTIONS

Start with a general warmup. Then, move on to the dumbbell exercises. Do 6 reps of exercise 2A, 6 reps of exercise 2B, 6 reps of exercise 2C, and so on, all the way down to exercise 2G. That's 1 set. Do a total of 3 sets of the "2" exercises.

1. Easy-Pace Row, Run, Bike, Stair-Climb: 10 Minutes

2A. Dumbbell Biceps Curl: 6 Reps

2B. Dumbbell Bent Row: 6 Reps

2C. Dumbbell Hang Clean: 6 Reps

2D. Dumbbell Front Squat Push Press: 6 Reps

2E. Dumbbell Overhead Squat: 6 Reps

2F. Pushup: 6 Reps

2G. Dumbbell Overhead Press: 6 Reps

Time: 15 to 20 Minutes

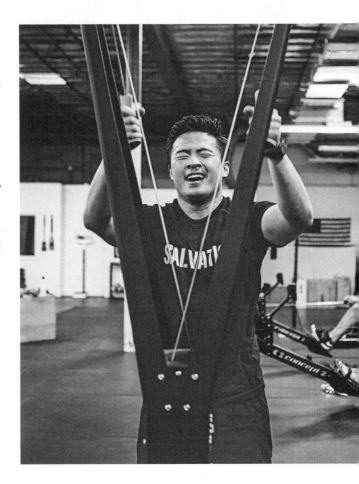

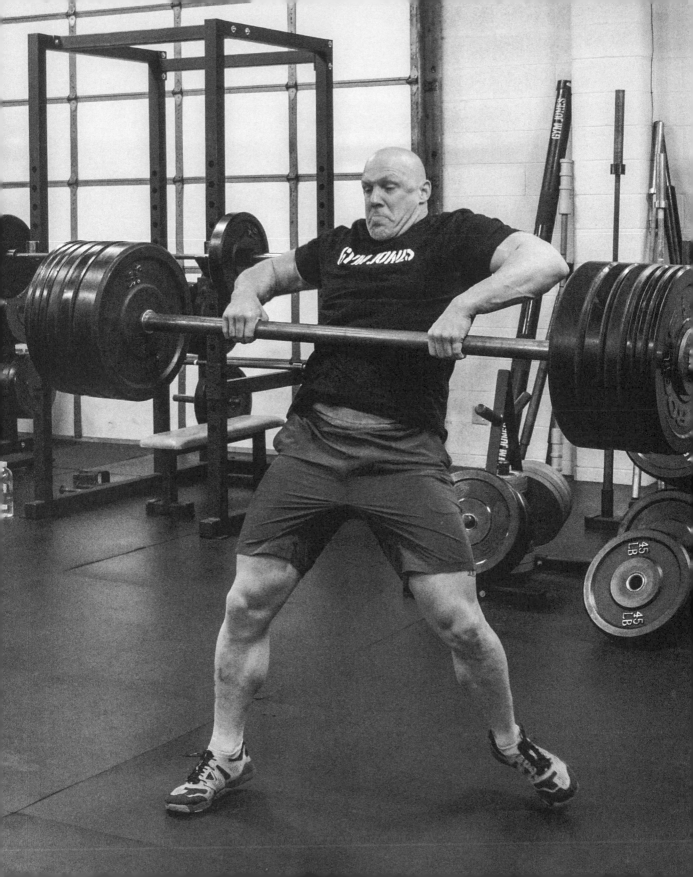

23

MAX TESTS

Knowing your 1-rep max will tell you exactly how strong you are in any given lift. That's critical for indicating where your fitness is and allowing you to determine where it needs to be. Once you know your 1-rep max (1RM), you'll know how heavy the weights should be for you to use in many of the workouts in this book.

DIRECTIONS

Determine which lift you're testing. Pick just one. Slowly add weight to the bar, doing just 1 rep with each successive weight until you find the heaviest weight that you can lift just 1 time with good form. During these testing workouts, you'll do anywhere from 10 to 25 single lifts. Warning: Don't perform these tests without capable spotters.

A common progression of adding weight may look like this:

▶ 135 pounds

▶ 155 pounds

▶ 185 pounds

▶ 205 pounds

▶ 225 pounds

▶ 245 pounds

▶ And so on, until you get to a point that you can no longer lift the weight.

Sets: As many as it takes to find the heaviest weight you can lift.

Time: 20 minutes

There are six different max tests you'll use in the program. The exercises, featured in the back, are:

Max Test 1: Barbell Bench Press
Max Test 2: Barbell Overhead Press
Max Test 3: Barbell Deadlift
Max Test 4: Barbell Front Squat
Max Test 5: Barbell Back Squat
Max Test 6: Barbell Overhead Squat

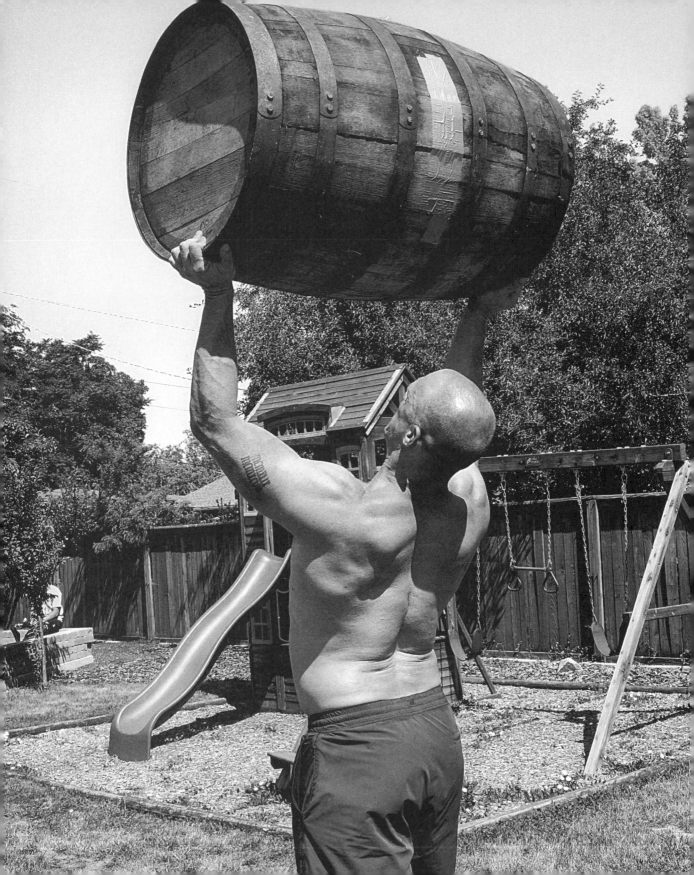

24

100 WORKOUTS

CIRCUIT-STYLE WORKOUTS

Circuit workouts include a series of exercises, performed in succession, using time to completion as the measure of performance. You rest, as needed, and your goal is to finish the workout as quickly as possible.

You'll find a few workouts in this section that don't follow that exact formula, which is why I decided to call this section "Circuit-Style" workouts. But every workout in this section delivers the same fitness effect on your body. Each leaves your muscles fatigued, works your cardiovascular system, and elevates your metabolism for 4 to 6 hours after training.

If you're familiar with fitness lingo, in this section, you'll find chippers, progressions, partner workouts, and a few other formats. Do each of the 25 workouts hard and with good form. My personal goal each time I train is to beat the time or the score I had before.

Bobby's Law:
In the real world, shit weighs what it weighs.

1

Circuit-Style 1
THE HOLY TRINITY

When I was fighting in the Ultimate Fighting Championship and working as a police officer, my time was extremely limited. I needed to pack high-level conditioning into a very short period of time—and so this body-weight workout was born. Prepare to do an incredible number of body-weight reps in just a half hour. That not only gives your muscles staying power, but it also boosts your cardiovascular fitness.

DIRECTIONS

Do 1 set of exercise 1, then 1 set of exercise 2, followed immediately by 1 set of exercise 3. That's 1 round. Do as many rounds as you can, resting as little as possible. Your goal is to do AMRAP (as many reps as possible) of each exercise in 30 minutes. Always use strict form. Some advice: Don't ever max out on a set, or you'll just blow up. In fact, if you can do, say, 30 pushups, 15 dips, and 10 pullups, you should probably do sets of about 5 to 10 pushups, 3 dips, and 2 or 3 pullups. A good goal to shoot for is 150 reps of each exercise.

1. Pushup

2. Pullup

3. Dip

Reps: AMRAP

Time: 30 Minutes

Circuit-Style 2
LOVE/HATE

I love the bench press. It's my favorite exercise of all time. One day, I went into the gym, and all I wanted to do was bench. The problem is that I firmly believe that you can't improve by only doing exercises that you love. So for a balanced workout, I decided to pair my bench presses with an exercise that I loathe: the burpee. After performing the workout, I found it was an excellent way to build serious upper-body strength while also logging some total-body, lung-taxing cardio. The result: a huge overall fitness benefit.

DIRECTIONS

In this workout, do the bench press with your body weight on the bar. So, if you weigh 185 pounds, the bar should weigh 185 pounds. (If that's too heavy, use the heaviest weight with which you can do 10 reps.) Then do burpees. It's designed in a digression/progression format, so do 10 reps of the bench press and 1 burpee, followed by 9 reps of the bench press and 2 burpees, 8 reps of the bench press and 3 burpees, and so on until you do 1 rep of the bench press and 10 burpees. Your goal is to complete the workout as fast as possible using good form. I've done it in 10 minutes and been destroyed afterward. You can also do it for fun, and take longer.

1. Barbell Bench Press: 10, 9, 8, 7, 6, 5, 4, 3, 2, 1 Reps

2. Burpee: 1, 2, 3, 4, 5, 6, 7, 8, 9, 10 Reps

Time: 10 to 20 Minutes

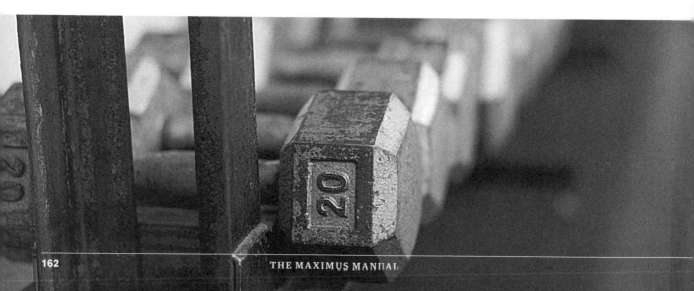

#3

Circuit-Style 3
400-METER MANSLAUGHTER

Salt Lake City is a beautiful city. The Wasatch Mountains provide a stunning backdrop no matter where in the city you are, and the weather is nice from spring to fall. On particularly nice days, I'll drag a few dumbbells or kettlebells to a track for a sunny, albeit difficult, training session. This workout packs in 400 reps each of a functional lower- and upper-body exercise. It takes about 25 minutes and makes you sore for days.

DIRECTIONS

Stand on the starting line of a track. Start by performing 5 reps of the dumbbell walking lunge (5 on each leg). Then, immediately do 5 push presses. Repeat until you've circled the track one time, which is 400 meters. Pro tip: Don't use too-heavy weights. I recommend 20 pounds for most guys.

1. Dumbbell Walking Lunge: 5 Reps

2. Dumbbell Push Press: 5 Reps

Distance: 400 Meters

Time: 25 Minutes

#4

Circuit-Style 4
FIVE FIFTY-FIVE

This is one of my all-time favorite workouts because it mixes heavy lifts and body-weight exercises and hits every muscle you have from head to toe. That gives you a training stimulus that builds real-world strength and muscle. Yes, it looks simple, but it's not—when you finish, you'll be "done," both figuratively and literally. It is adapted from a workout by a strength and conditioning coach I greatly admire, Dan John.

DIRECTIONS

Do the exercises in order, as a circuit. Do 10 reps of the first exercise, 10 reps of the next, and so on, until you've completed all of the exercises. Then repeat the circuit, this time doing 9 reps of each. Repeat the circuit again, doing 8 reps of each, then 7 reps of each, and so on until you do only 1 rep of each exercise. Rest as needed throughout, and try to complete the workout as quickly as possible, while maintaining good form. Beginners can use a 95-pound barbell; intermediates can use a 185-pound barbell; and advanced trainees can use a 225-pound barbell.

1. Barbell Bench Press

2. Barbell Deadlift

3. Pushup

4. Pullup

5. Barbell Back Squat

Reps: 10-9-8-7-6-5-4-3-2-1 of Each

Time: 15 to 25 Minutes

#5

Circuit-Style 5
WELCOME PARTY

This workout is your welcome to the gym. It takes only 5 minutes and anyone can do it, but what I'm looking for is whether you truly go all out—Welcome Party is a test of your psychological willpower more than anything else. If you go hard enough, you're invited to stay and train with me. If you slack off, you're invited to leave.

DIRECTIONS

Load a barbell so it weighs 135 pounds. Start by doing 20 barbell bench presses, then do 20 burpee pullups. If you can't do 20 consecutive reps of one or both of the exercises, simply rest, as needed, during each set until you can finish. Then, immediately do 10 barbell bench presses followed by 10 burpee pullups.

1. Barbell Bench Press
2. Burpee Pullup

Reps: 20, 10 of Each
Time: 3 to 5 Minutes

#6

Circuit-Style 6
GUT PUNCH

The quickest way to a six-pack isn't lying on your back doing situps, it's doing this workout. The Gut Punch hammers your entire lower body—your strongest muscles—and also your entire core. Use strict form and work hard, and your core will be so sore that you may not want to laugh for a week.

DIRECTIONS

Grab two 16-kilogram kettlebells or 35-pound dumbbells, and do 50 reps of the stepup (25 on each leg). Then do 50 reps of feet-to-hands. (If that exercise is too advanced, do knees-to-elbows instead.) Repeat, this time doing 40 reps of each. Now repeat three more times, doing 30, 20, and 10 reps, respectively.

1. Dumbbell/Kettlebell Stepup
2. Feet-to-Hands (or Knees-to-Elbows)

Reps: 50, 40, 30, 20, 10 of Each
Time: 15 to 25 Minutes

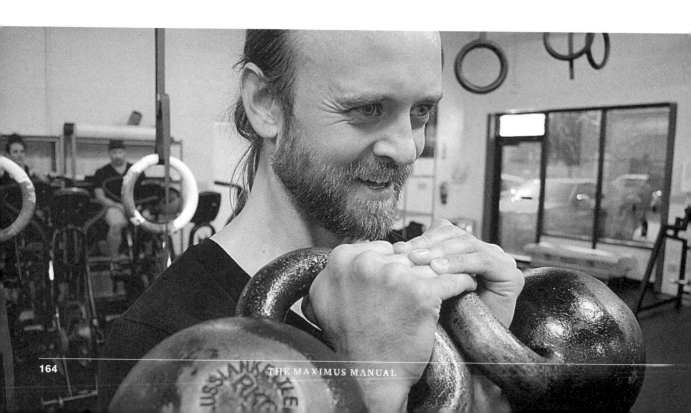

#7

Circuit-Style 7
CIRCUS MAXIMUS

I'm a huge fan of workouts that absolutely crush you in less than 25 minutes. By the end of this one, you'll feel like you've just lost a gladiator battle. Despite the fact that everyone absolutely hates it, Circus Maximus is so effective that the guys at the gym have been doing this workout for as long as I can remember.

DIRECTIONS

Do the workout as a circuit. Start with the dumbbell front squat push press (use 30-pound dumbbells), then do the pushups, followed by the deadlifts (use a 135-pound barbell). That's 1 round. Do 12 rounds.

1. Dumbbell Front Squat Push Press: 12 Reps

2. Pushup: 12 Reps

3. Barbell Deadlift: 12 Reps

Rounds: 12
Time: 15 to 25 Minutes

#8

Circuit-Style 8
MY COMPLIMENTS

A complementary circuit is a circuit that uses two or more opposing muscle groups. You might, for example, pair lower-body and upper-body exercises, or push and pull movements. When one muscle group is working, the other rests, which allows you to work harder in the circuit and stress your cardiovascular system more.

DIRECTIONS

Load a bar with a weight equal to about 125 percent of your body weight. So, for example, if you weigh 200 pounds, your bar would weigh 250. Start with 30 deadlifts. Then, do 30 handstand pushups. (If those are too advanced, do regular pushups.) That's 1 round. Repeat, this time doing 20 reps of both exercises, followed by 10 reps, for a total of 3 rounds.

1. Barbell Deadlift

2. Handstand Pushup (or Pushup)

Reps: 30, 20, 10 of Each
Rounds: 3
Time: 10 to 25 Minutes

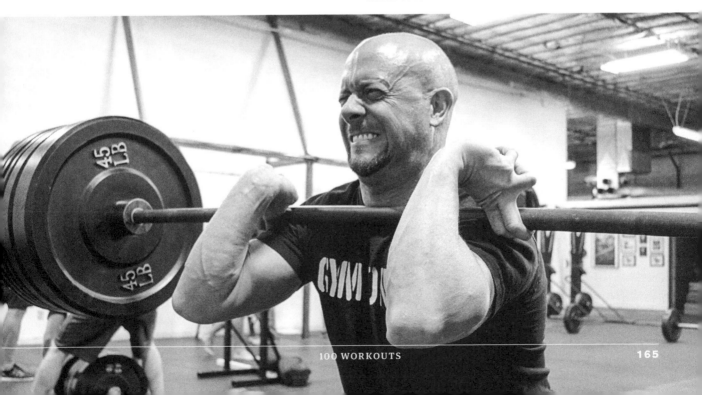

Circuit-Style 9
OPPOSITES ATTRACT

This workout puts you through the wringer. Like "Circuit-Style 8: My Compliments," it's also a complementary circuit, so your goal is to finish fast. But because it's a longer workout with lighter weights, there's more of a cardiovascular effect. Prepare to feel like your lungs are engulfed in flames.

DIRECTIONS

Load a bar with a weight equal to your body weight. Start with the deadlifts and do 15 reps. Then, move on to the bench press—I suggest using 135 pounds (or do regular pushups if that's too heavy)—and do 15 reps. That's 1 round. Do 5 rounds, resting as little as possible.

1. Barbell Deadlift: 15 Reps
2. Barbell Bench Press (or Pushup): 15 Reps

Rounds: 5
Time: 5 to 10 Minutes

10

Circuit-Style 10
DON'T ASK ME ABOUT YOUR ABS

Don't tell me you want to do an "abs workout." The truth is that when you train with the exercises in this book, your core is always activated. So, by default, any routine gives your abs a workout. I give this brutal workout to people who ask to devote an entire session to doing an abs workout—it ensures that they never ask me again. Your abs will be sore for days.

DIRECTIONS

Perform the exercises as a circuit. Start with the first exercise, and do it for 30 seconds. Then "rest" for 30 seconds, but as you do, perform 5 pushups. Move onto the next exercise for 30 seconds, followed again by 30 seconds of rest that includes 5 pushups. Repeat the pattern until you've done all the exercises. That's 1 round. Do a total of 3 rounds.

1. Situp
2. Pushup Position Plank
3. V-Sit Kickout
4. V-Sit Hold
5. Leg Raise
6. Leg Raise Hold
7. Feet-to-Hands
8. Pushup Position Plank

Work: 30 Seconds
Rest: 30 Seconds with 5 Pushups
Rounds: 3
Time: 24 Minutes

#11

Circuit-Style 11
EDIMFSD

Because your shoulders are involved in any exercise where you hold a weight, I like to say that "every day is motherf*ing shoulder day." But with this workout, that's especially true. Holding weight above your head not only fatigues your shoulders, but also works on your mobility, stability, and your core.

DIRECTIONS

Do the workout as a circuit. Start with 30 overhead squats. Use a bar that weighs 35 percent of your body weight. So if you weigh 200 pounds, your bar would weigh 70 pounds. Then, do 30 reps of the bench press using 135 pounds. (If that's too heavy, just do regular pushups instead.) Repeat, this time doing 20 reps of both exercises, and then 10 reps. Rest as little as possible.

1. Barbell Overhead Squat
2. Barbell Bench Press (or Pushup)

Reps: 30, 20, 10 of Each
Time: 5 to 10 Minutes

#12

Circuit-Style 12
BALLS TO THE WALLS

This was my very first introduction to circuit training, and it left me crippled. I'd never seen or felt anything like it. Afterward, my leg muscles were so filled with lactic acid that I couldn't see any definition, and I was sore for a week. I was hooked and never looked back.

DIRECTIONS

Grab a 20-pound medicine ball. Do 50 wall balls, then 50 ball slams. Repeat, but this time do 40 reps of each. Repeat 3 more times, doing 30, 20, and 10 reps, respectively, resting as little as possible.

1. Wall Ball
2. Ball Slam

Reps: 50, 40, 30, 20, 10 of Each
Time: 10 to 20 Minutes

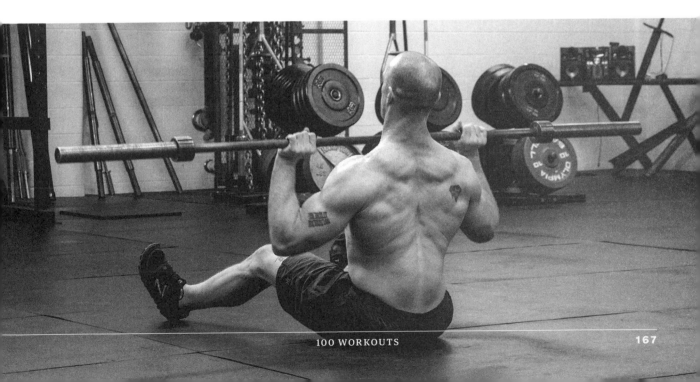

#13

Circuit-Style 13
THE DISTANCE

In boxing, going "the distance" means that you fought through every round of a fight, 12 full rounds, if it's a championship fight. I've done it, and by the opening bell of the last round your legs feel like rubber and you can barely stand. If you do this workout as quickly as possible, you'll feel the same as you enter the final round. Then it's up to you to decide whether to answer the bell or throw in the towel.

DIRECTIONS

Load a bar with 225 pounds (it's okay to use less weight if you can't deadlift 225 pounds 10 times). Do 10 deadlifts. Then do 25 box jumps onto a 24-inch box. That's 1 round. Do a total of 3 rounds, resting as little as possible.

1. Barbell Deadlift: 10 Reps
2. Box Jump: 25 Reps

Rounds: 3
Time: 5 to 7 Minutes

#14

Circuit-Style 14
1775

I consider it a true honor that the US government hires me to train its elite soldiers. I've had the opportunity to work with many marines during my career, and I believe these men should be celebrated. The rep scheme, 17 and 75, celebrates the year the US Marine Corps was founded, 1775. There are 4 rounds: 1 for God, 1 for country, 1 for The Corps, and 1 for Chesty Puller, the most decorated marine in history. I do this version of the workout every November 10, the day of the Marine Corps' birthday. Do it right, and once a year is enough.

DIRECTIONS

Do 17 burpee pullups, then do 75 lunges. That's 1 round. Do 4 rounds, resting only as needed.

1. Burpee Pullup: 17 Reps
2. Lunge: 75 Reps

Rounds: 4
Time: 10 to 20 Minutes

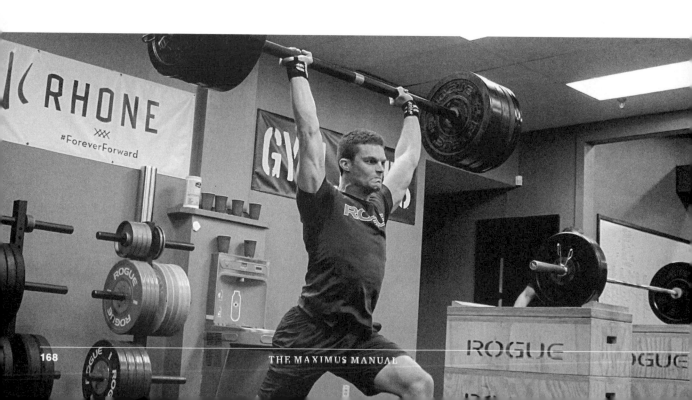

#15

Cirouit-Style 15
LOAD AND EXPLODE

Want to crush your legs? This is your ticket. The workout pairs explosive split jumps and grinding deadlifts. The key is to make your split jumps as explosive as possible: If you're not trying to launch your body into the roof of the gym every rep, you're only cheating yourself.

DIRECTIONS

Load a bar with 80 percent of your 1-rep max deadlift. If you can deadlift 350 pounds, for example, use a bar weighing 280 pounds. Do 5 deadlifts. Then, do 20 split jumps, 10 on each leg. That's 1 round. Do a total of 5 rounds, resting as little as possible.

1. Barbell Deadlift: 5 Reps

2. Split Jump: 20 Reps

Rounds: 5
Time: 5 to 10 Minutes

#16

Circuit-Style 16
THE BEST FOR LAST

Prepare to experience firsthand why burpees suck. At first, you'll think that you're breezing through the workout. Then, you'll reach the burpees, a point where all time and space seems to stall—that section of the workout feels like a black hole you'll never escape from. Indeed, 70 burpees is about 60 too many.

DIRECTIONS

Do the exercises in the order shown. Complete all the prescribed reps of movement, then move on to the next exercise, resting as little as possible. Once you complete the final exercise, you're done. Use two 20-pound dumbbells for the dumbbell front squat push presses, and a 24-inch box for the box jumps.

1. Pullup: 20 Reps

2. Dumbbell Front Squat Push Press: 30 Reps

3. Box Jump: 40 Reps

4. Pushup: 50 Reps

5. Situp: 60 Reps

6. Burpee: 70 Reps

Time: 10 to 15 Minutes

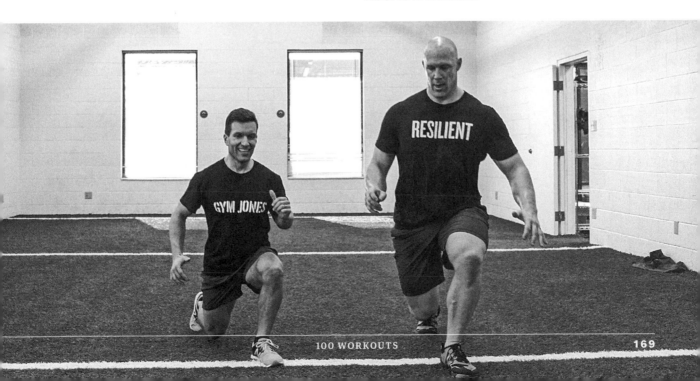

#17

Circuit-Style 17
SUPERHERO

Besides superpowers, what do all superheroes have in common? Broad, strong shoulders. This workout is one of my favorite ways to build those type of shoulders. In this workout, most people try to lower their times by using shoddy form on the handstand pushups and pullups. Keep them strict, and take a little longer to do the circuit.

DIRECTIONS

Do the exercises in the order shown. Complete all the prescribed reps of movement, then move on to the next exercise, resting as little as possible. Once you complete the final exercise, you're done. Use a barbell weighing the equivalent of your body weight for the barbell bench presses, and a 24-kilogram kettlebell for the kettlebell swing. If you can't do strict handstand pushups, which is common, do dumbbell or barbell overhead presses instead.

1. **Handstand Pushup (or Dumbbell or Barbell Overhead Press):** 25 Reps
2. **Barbell Bench Press:** 35 Reps
3. **Pullup:** 45 Reps
4. **Kettlebell Swing:** 55 Reps
5. **Situp:** 65 Reps
6. **Burpee:** 75 Reps

Time: 10 to 30 Minutes

#18

Circuit-Style 18
IT'S TRICKY

When I write this on the workout board, people always think that their legs are going to take the brunt of the hammering. I get it. There are six squat variations totaling 250 reps. But, once you get cranking, your core will wear down far faster than your legs. That's because exercises like the overhead squat, front squat, and back squat all require you to lock down your core, and they're each followed by a direct core exercise. Think of this one as a workout for every muscle you have from your pecs down.

DIRECTIONS

Do the exercises in the order shown. Complete all the prescribed reps of movement, then move on to the next exercise, resting as little as possible. Once you complete the final exercise, you're done. Try to use a 45-pound bar for the overhead squats, a 95-pound bar for the front squats, a 135-pound bar for the back squats, and a 70-pound dumbbell for the goblet squats.

1. **Barbell Overhead Squat:** 20 Reps
2. **Feet-to-Hands:** 20 Reps
3. **Barbell Front Squat:** 30 Reps
4. **Knees-to-Elbows:** 30 Reps
5. **Barbell Back Squat:** 40 Reps
6. **V-Sit Kickout:** 40 Reps
7. **Goblet Squat:** 50 Reps
8. **Air Squat:** 50 Reps
9. **Squat:** 60 Reps
10. **Curlup:** 60 Reps

Time: 20 to 30 Minutes

#19

Circuit-Style 19
MEANT TO MOVE

Jumping and stepping are arguably the two most functional movements. Done intensely as a workout, they make for a routine that's far more transferable to the real world than something like the elliptical. What's more, you can generally see a better cardio effect—the key is to push the pace on the steps and jumps. Try to log as many reps as possible in each round. If you do it right, this can be one of the hardest workouts you'll ever do.

DIRECTIONS

Do box jumps onto a 20-inch box for 30 seconds. Immediately do body-weight stepups for 60 seconds onto the same box. Rest for 30 seconds. That's 1 round. Do a total of 14 rounds.

1. **Box Jump:** 30 Seconds
2. **Stepup:** 60 Seconds
3. **Rest:** 30 Seconds

Rounds: 14
Time: 28 Minutes

#20

Circuit-Style 20
IT'S A DEEP BURN

The name doesn't lie. Performing 300 reps straight, as fast as possible, creates an incredible amount of acidity in your legs. People who go through this without rest often have difficulty walking for days. I've also seen people take it easier, break up the reps, and go slowly to concentrate on form, but they also have difficulty walking for a few days. Hell, any way you do it, your legs are going to be sore, but you're going to be better for it.

DIRECTIONS

Grab a 24-inch box, two 25-pound dumbbells, and a 20-pound medicine ball. Do 100 box jumps, then 100 dumbbell front squat push presses, then 100 wall balls. No more, no less.

1. **Box Jump:** 100 Reps
2. **Dumbbell Front Squat Push Press:** 100 Reps
3. **Wall Ball:** 100 Reps

Time: 10 to 20 Minutes

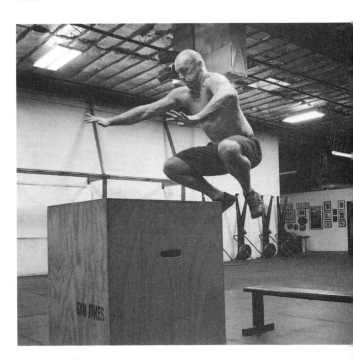

#21

Circuit-Style 21
SORE LEGS, NO EQUIPMENT

This workout doesn't require a single piece of equipment, but it's an incredible lower-body workout. In fact, it's my go-to when I'm stuck somewhere, like a hotel, that doesn't have a good gym. Think of it as basically 30 minutes of your legs screaming at you.

DIRECTIONS

Do 40 alternating lunges, 20 on each leg. Then do a wall sit for 30 seconds. Then do 38 lunges (19 on each leg), followed again by a 30-second wall sit. Then, do 36 lunges (18 on each leg), followed by a 30-second wall sit. Follow that pattern of doing 1 less lunge on each leg followed by a 30-second wall sit until you've done just 1 lunge on each leg. Try to make it through the workout without resting.

1. Lunge: 40, 38, 36, 34 . . . 6, 4, 2, 1 Reps
2. Wall Sit: 30 Seconds

Rounds: 20, Done in Digression Format
Time: 20 to 25 Minutes

#22

Circuit-Style 22
GRIND/EXPLODE

Pairing heavy squats with explosive jumps elicits what scientists call a postactivation potentiation effect. It allows you to recruit more motor neurons, which then enables you to jump higher, and, therefore, improve your fitness. The key is to jump as high as possible on each split jump. Lazy jumps lead to lazy legs. Work hard and build yourself the set of wheels you deserve.

DIRECTIONS

Grab a 24-kilogram kettlebell or a 55-pound dumbbell. Do 10 goblet squats, followed by 20 split jumps (10 on each leg). Rest for 2 minutes. That's 1 round. Do a total of 10 rounds.

1. Goblet Squat: 10 Reps
2. Split Jump: 20 Reps
3. Rest: 2 Minutes

Rounds: 10
Time: 30 Minutes

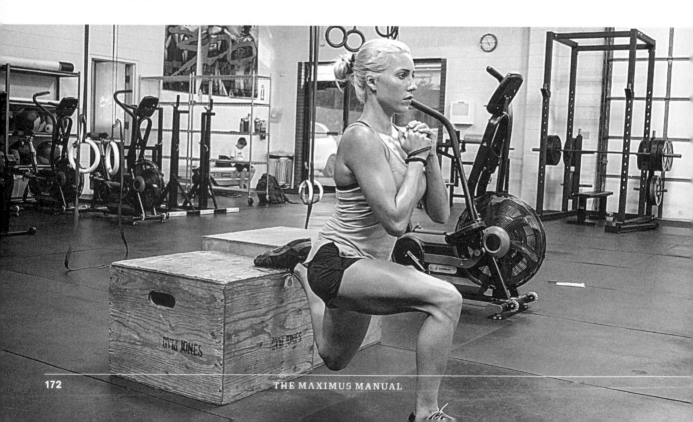

Circuit-Style 23
THE MAXIMUS 500

If there was just one workout that would give you "The Maximus Body," this 500-rep nightmare is it. In it, you do my favorite exercises of all time at a rapid pace. You work your entire body, and your heart rate goes through the roof, so you see incredible strength- and muscle-building and fat-burning effects. Focus on finishing this workout as quickly as you can while maintaining excellent technique. I'll often do this workout both before and after a fitness program to help me determine just how much I've improved. Do the same: Keep track of your times, and try to improve each time you do it.

DIRECTIONS

Perform the exercises in the order shown. Complete all the prescribed reps of the first exercise, then move on to the next exercise, resting as little as possible. Once you complete the final exercise, you're done. Try to use a 65-pound barbell for the strict press, a 24-kilogram kettlebell for the goblet squat, a 135-pound bar for the deadlifts, back squats, and bench press, and a 24-inch box for the box jumps.

1. Pullup: 50 Reps

2. Barbell Back Squat: 50 Reps

3. Barbell Deadlift: 50 Reps

4. Goblet Squat: 50 Reps

5. Barbell Bench Press: 50 Reps

6. Strict Press: 50 Reps

7. Pushup: 50 Reps

8. Ball Slam: 50 Reps

9. Box Jump: 50 Reps

10. Burpee: 50 Reps

Time: 15 to 30 Minutes

Circuit-Style 24
ALTITUDE ADJUSTMENT

For the past 9 years, I've lived in Salt Lake City, Utah—a town that's about 4,300 feet above sea level. Before people visit, they routinely ask me how to train to prepare for the altitude. I give them this workout. Do it right, and it'll feel like the oxygen in the room has completely disappeared. You can do it with a partner, or you can do it alone.

DIRECTIONS

If you have two people, one person runs 400 meters as fast as possible. As he does, the other person holds two 24-kilogram kettlebells in the rack position. Once the first person finishes running 400 meters, the two people immediately switch positions. When the second person finishes his 400 meters, that's 1 round. Don't rest. Immediately repeat until you've finished 5 rounds. The faster you run, the less time your partner has to spend under the weight of the kettlebells. If you don't have a partner, that's no problem. Just hold the kettlebells the amount of time it took you to run the 400 meters. If the first run takes you 70 seconds, for example, then hold the kettlebells for 70 seconds. If the second run takes you 90 seconds, then hold the kettlebells for 90 seconds.

1. Run: 400 Meters

2. Kettlebell Rack Hold: For 400-Meter Run Time

Rounds: 5
Time: 10 to 20 Minutes

#25

Circuit-Style 25
MAXIMUS WEDDING WORKOUT

When I got married in July of 2016, it wasn't just a celebration of love. It was also a celebration of the community I've built. Instructors I've certified flew in from around the country, and, after the wedding, we all did this workout. You can do it with a partner, like we all did, or you can do it alone. We were married on July 3 (07/03), which is why there are 7 exercises in the circuit, and you do 3 total rounds. This turned out to be one of my favorite workouts ever, not only because of the meaning behind it but also because it's surprisingly difficult.

DIRECTIONS

Do the exercises in the order shown. Do each exercise for 30 seconds, rest for 30 seconds, then move on to the next exercise, and repeat. Once you've completed all 7 exercises, that's 1 round. Do a total of 3 rounds.

1. **Frog Hop**
2. **Pushup**
3. **Split Jump**
4. **Burpee**
5. **Squat**
6. **Squat Hold**
7. **Situp**

Work: 30 Seconds
Rest: 30 Seconds
Rounds: 3
Time: 21 Minutes

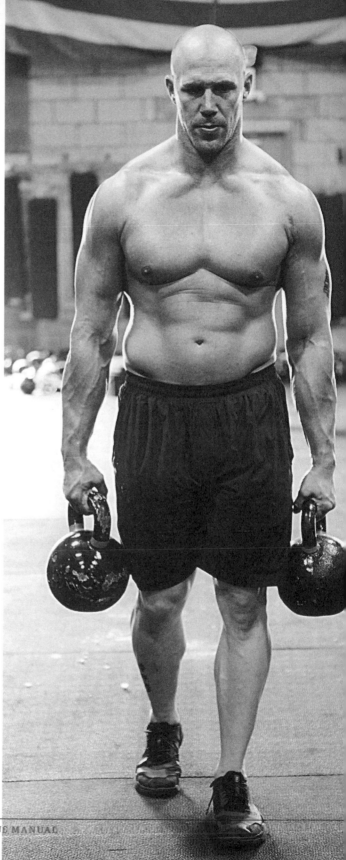

"DEATH BY" WORKOUTS

I live for "Death By" workouts. Before I explain why I love them so much, let me explain their simple premise. You pick one exercise and set a timer. The first minute, you do 1 rep of the exercise. The second minute, you do 2 reps of the exercise, the third minute, 3 reps, and so on. When you can't finish your reps—say, 20 reps on minute 20—the workout ends.

These workouts are simple, but not easy. They teach you to push yourself to the limit and to put yourself in an uncomfortable position. They also kill your excuses, because they require minimal equipment and time. In fact, most take less than 20 minutes, and require only a will to suffer.

The first 5 minutes will seem easy. But after minute six, the fun stops, and they become a mental crucible. The first moment when your brain tells you it's time to stop, you need to recognize that you still have at least 2 more minutes in you. Pushing and getting that extra 2 minutes is where the real magic happens.

In this section, I listed my five favorite "Death By" workouts, but you can also use your imagination and create your own. Pick an exercise and go. Depending on the movement, you may last 10 minutes, or you may last 30. To find what you're looking for, all you have to do is go hard.

#26

1. Death by
BURPEE

This workout is particularly great at forcing you to face what I call the "moment," that special point in a workout where you cave in to your mental demons and quit, or overcome, continue pushing, and finish mentally and physically stronger.

DIRECTIONS
Start a timer, and do 1 burpee during minute one. Do 2 burpees during minute two, 3 burpees during minute three, and so on, until you're all out of burpees

1. Burpee

Rounds: As Many As Possible
Time: 10 to 20 Minutes

#27

2. Death by
10 METERS

Running is a natural human movement. We're bipedal creatures, and we're built to move on our feet for extended periods of time. There's nothing better than running for developing your overall cardiovascular function.

DIRECTIONS
Start a timer, and run 10 meters during minute one. Run 20 meters during minute two, run 30 meters during minute three, and so on, until you can't complete all your meters.

Not sure how long 10 meters is? Just take 10 giant steps, and you'll be close enough. Note: This workout is meant to be done as a shuttle run. Measure off 10 meters and run back and forth to complete your desired distance. Pro tip: Go easy during your first handful of sprints, or you'll blow up early.

1. 10-Meter Sprint

Rounds: As Many As Possible
Time: 15 to 25 Minutes

28

3. Death by
PUSHUP

Most people look at these "Death By" workouts and say that they don't allow for enough reps. Here's a stat to counter that argument: 465. That's how many pushups you'd do if you got to minute 30 of this workout. When's the last time you did 465 pushups in half an hour? Probably never.

DIRECTIONS

Start a timer, and do 1 pushup during minute one. Do 2 pushups during minute two, 3 pushups during minute three, and so on, until you're all out of pushups.

1. Pushup

Rounds: As Many As Possible
Time: 10 to 30 Minutes

29

4. Death by
AIR SQUAT

This is probably the most deceptive workout I've ever done. I mean, how hard is it to do one squat in 1 minute or even 10 squats in a minute? Soon enough, though, you're at minute 20, 30, or 40, and the sheer volume of reps absolutely overwhelms you. I've seen people make it to round 45, which is 1,035 total squats. May God have mercy on your sore legs.

DIRECTIONS

Start a timer, and do 1 air squat during minute one. Do 2 air squats during minute two, 3 air squats during minute three, and so on, until you're all out of air squats.

1. Air Squat

Rounds: As Many As Possible
Time: 15 to 45 Minutes

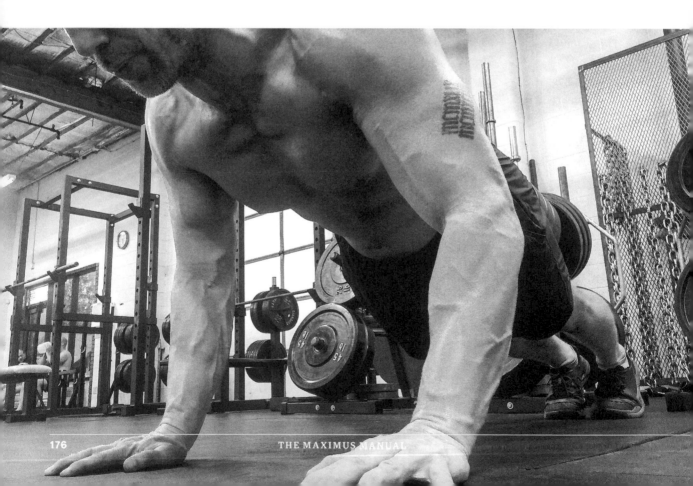

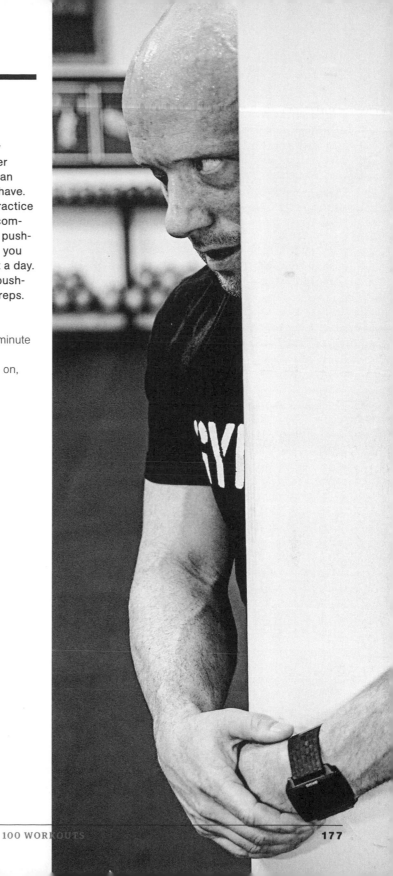

#30

5. Death by
HANDSTAND PUSHUP

Handstand pushups challenge your upper-body strength and stability more than nearly any other exercise. Learning to do them with good form can correct many shoulder or core issues you may have. That's why I use this workout most often as a practice session for improving my handstand pushups, compared to using it as a burner. Do the handstand pushups strict—shoot for form instead of reps. Once you reach 10 rounds and accumulate 55 reps, call it a day. If you can't do handstand pushups, do regular pushups, focusing on good form over accumulating reps.

DIRECTIONS

Start a timer, and do 1 handstand pushup during minute one. Do 2 handstand pushups during minute two, 3 handstand pushups during minute three, and so on, until you reach minute 10.

1. Handstand Pushup

Rounds: As Many As Possible, Stopping at 10
Time: 5 to 10 Minutes

III. INTERVAL WORKOUTS

Interval training is the best way to increase your endurance quickly. In these workouts, you do an incredibly intense bout of work, followed by a rest period. The reason this structure works at boosting your endurance is because resting allows you to regroup, and then to give a maximum effort again. That way, you accumulate more time at the highest exercise intensities.

Most of these workouts are done on a row machine, bike, or ski ergometer—or you simply run—but you can choose any cardio machine you want. The machine means nothing compared to your effort—effort is key. In fact, I've done these workouts on everything from an elliptical trainer (when stuck in a hotel) to a climbing machine (that was a very bad day), to a classic stair-stepper.

I ask people to aim for 90- to 95-percent effort on each interval. I always require them to get better or faster each time they do the same workout.

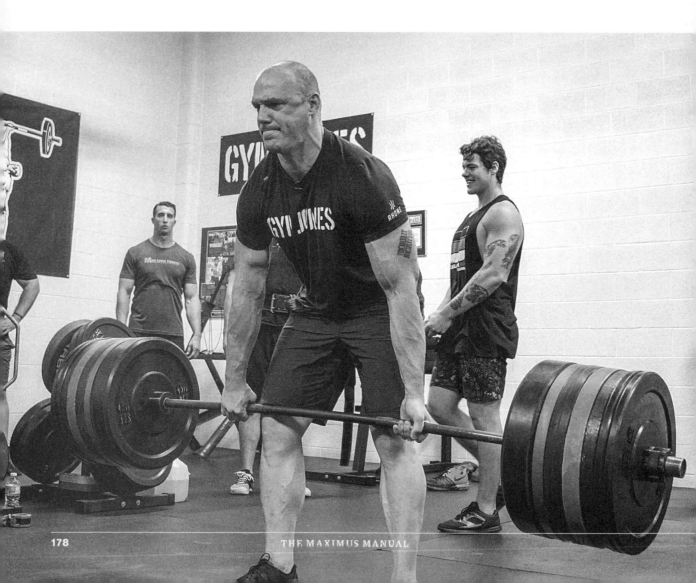

#31

Interval 1
30/30

My two favorite pieces of cardio equipment are the rowing machine and the ski ergometer. Both are relatively inexpensive (under $1,000), and they're absolutely bomb-proof. That's why, if you're going to buy a cardio machine for your home, I recommend one of these two. Most gyms have a rower, and I see more and more ski ergometers. (If your gym doesn't have either, you can run on a treadmill or ride an exercise bike for this workout.) It ramps up your cardiovascular output, so you can go faster and longer in endurance events, and can better handle high-intensity lifting days.

DIRECTIONS

Row, ski, or run as hard as you can for 30 seconds. Then rest for 30 seconds. That's 1 round. Do 6 total rounds, and then rest for 4 minutes straight. That's 1 block. Do 3 total blocks. Beginners should aim to row or ski 150 meters each round, while intermediates should hit 160, and advanced trainees should log 170.

1. Row, Ski, or Run

Work: 30 Seconds
Rest: 30 Seconds between Rounds, 4 Minutes between Blocks
Blocks: 3, Comprised of 6 Rounds Each (18 Total Rounds)
Time: 30 Minutes

#32

Interval 2
500-METER MURDER

I love the 500-meter row distance because it allows you to build your endurance and your power. Your lungs need to be efficient enough so that you don't gas out, but your muscles also have to be strong enough to rocket you through the meters as fast as possible. (If you don't have access to a rower or ski ergometer, you can also run or ride an exercise bike as hard as possible for about 1:45 each round.) In this workout, I ask that you finish your 500 meters faster each succeeding round. That not only helps improve your fitness but also it keeps you from slacking off in later rounds, which builds mental strength.

DIRECTIONS

Set a rower or ski ergometer's computer for 500 meters. Begin, trying to finish the row about 15 seconds slower than your 500-meter PR (personal record) pace. For example, if the fastest 500-meter you've ever rowed took you 1:30, your first round of this workout should take you about 1:45. Rest for 2 minutes. That's 1 round. Repeat, trying to finish each successive round even faster. On your fifth and final round, you should go all out, finishing as fast as you can.

1. Row or Ski: 500 Meters
2. Rest: 2 Minutes

Rounds: 5
Time: 20 Minutes

#33

Interval 3
FAN BIKE TO HELL

If you do it right, this may be the hardest workout in this book. In it, you burn 50 calories on a fan bike, then 40, then 30, then 20, and then 10. Because of the bike's fan and the nature of wind resistance, the harder you pedal, the harder pedaling becomes—the bike almost fights back. So, how do you do this workout "right"? Go as hard as you possibly can each ride. That's actually a requirement with the people I train, but this workout is so sinister that even my most dedicated athletes sometimes secretly try to pace themselves. Good luck.

DIRECTIONS

Hop on a fan bike (if you don't have a fan bike, try burpees for reps or try rowing for calories, as in "Interval 4: Row to Hell" at right), and set its computer so it's measuring your calorie burn. Ride as hard as you possibly can until you hit 50 calories. Rest as long as it took you to complete your 50-calorie ride. So, for example, if you burned 50 calories in 1 minute, you'd rest for 1 minute. Next, repeat for 40 calories, resting afterward for the amount of time it took you to burn those 40 calories. Continue to repeat the pattern until you do your final 10-calorie sprint. Note: This workout is also fun to do with a partner, following the "you go, I go," format, where you ride, then rest as your partner rides.

1. Fan Bike: Burn 50, 40, 30, 20, 10 Calories Digressively

2. Rest: Time It Took to Complete Last Effort

Rounds: 5
Time: 10 to 20 Minutes

#34

Interval 4
ROW TO HELL

This workout is like "Fan Bike to Hell," except that you start with 500 meters and work your way down—100 meters at a time—until you row just 100 meters. Row to Hell is slightly less intense, but it also takes longer to complete, which is why it delivers a better cardio effect. Suffer more intensely with the "Fan Bike to Hell," or suffer longer with "Row to Hell"—it's up to you.

DIRECTIONS

Hop on a row machine and set its computer so it's measuring your meters rowed. Row as hard as you possibly can until you hit 500 meters. (If you don't have a row machine, you can also use a ski ergometer or a fan bike.) Rest as long as it took you to complete your 500-meter row. So, for example, if you rowed 500 meters in 1:30, you'd rest for 1:30. Repeat for 400 meters this time, resting afterward for the amount of time it took you to row those 400 meters. Repeat the pattern until you do your final 100-meter row. Note: This workout is also fun to do with a partner, following the "you go, I go," format, where you row, then rest as your partner rows.

1. Row: To Cover 500, 400, 300, 200, 100 Meters Digressively

2. Rest: Time It Took to Complete Last Distance

Rounds: 5
Time: 15 to 25 Minutes

#35

Interval 5
LET'S MAKE A DEAL

In this workout, you and I are going to make a bargain, which I'm hoping will make you work harder: You're going to row or ski for 2,000 meters. If you log a personal record on that challenge, you're done. If you don't, then you have to row or ski for 1,000 meters, then another 500 meters. Having a reward—even when the payoff is not having to do more exercise—is a great way to trick yourself into pushing harder.

DIRECTIONS

Row or ski 2,000 meters as fast as possible. If you don't achieve your fastest 2,000-meter time ever, rest for the amount of time it took you to complete 2,000 meters. For example, if your row lasted 7 minutes, rest for 7 minutes. Then, row 1,000 meters. Rest for the time it took you to complete 1,000 meters. Then, row 500 meters.

1. Row or Ski: 2,000 Meters

2. If no PR, Rest for Time Equal to Complete 2,000 Meters

3. Row or Ski: 1,000 Meters

4. Rest for Time Equal to Complete 1,000 Meters

5. Row or Ski: 500 Meters

Time: 30 Minutes

#36

Interval 6
THE LONG ROAD

As I mentioned in the first section of this book, the key to building a big base of endurance is keeping your heart rate elevated for an extended period of time. This is one of the longer interval workouts in this book. Like most interval workouts, it jacks up your heart rate so you'll improve your ability to go all out, but it also keeps your heart rate high longer than usual, so you'll see a massive cardiovascular benefit.

DIRECTIONS

Row or ski 500 meters in 2 minutes. Rest for 1 minute. That's 1 round. Do 10 total rounds, trying to take 1 or 2 seconds off your time each round. So, for example, you'd want to finish your second round in 1:59, and your last round somewhere around 1:45. If you don't have access to a rower or ski ergometer, you can also do this outside by running around a track one-and-a-half times (600 meters).

1. Row or Ski: 500 Meters (or Run: 600 Meters)

2. Rest: 1 Minute between Rounds

Rounds: 10

Time: 30 Minutes

37

Interval 7
ADD A METER

Pacing is the key to setting a personal record in any cardiovascular event. If you go too hard too early, you'll only blow up and fall short. That's why, when I was training to break the ski ergometer 500-meter world record, I did many of these workouts. In them, you're tasked with rowing or skiing a certain distance each round. Each successive round, your new goal becomes your last round's distance plus one. Go too hard, and you'll keep building up meters until your final rounds are absolutely hellish. For example, if my goal distance is 150 meters, nailing it exactly means that the next round I go 151 meters. But, if I actually ski 157 meters, my next goal is 158. That a built-in penalty for overexertion teaches you to pace yourself.

DIRECTIONS

Set the rower or ski ergometer, using the intervals/time function, to 30 seconds work and 1:30 of rest. Row or ski 150 meters in 30 seconds. Rest for 1 minute and 30 seconds. That's 1 round. Do 15 rounds, trying to go 1 more meter than your last round. So, for example, your second round you might go 151 meters, and your third would be 152. The catch: If you go more than the prescribed meters on any one round, you have to go up by 1 meter from that number your next round.

1. Row or Ski: 30 Seconds

2. Rest: 90 Seconds

Rounds: 15
Time: 30 Minutes

38

Interval 8
WHEELS

Some strength and conditioning trainers bash running. But my opinion is that if you can't cover ground fast, you're not really that fit. Running is a natural human movement that's the easiest way to improve your heart strength. One of my favorite speed distances is 800 meters, which is just about half a mile. It's the perfect distance to challenge your brain as well as your body.

DIRECTIONS

Run 800 meters (0.5 mile) at your 2-mile personal best pace (see "Max Tests" on page 159). If your fastest 2-mile run took you 14 minutes, for example, then each 800-meter, or half-mile, run should take you about 3:30. Rest for the same amount of time it takes you to run the 800. So in the above example, you'd rest for 3:30. That's 1 round. Do a total of 7 rounds.

1. Run: 800 meters (0.5 mile)

2. Rest: Time to Complete Distance

Rounds: 7
Time: 45 Minutes

#39

Interval 9
TABATA TRIPLETS

In 1996, a Japanese scientist named Izumi Tabata changed the fitness industry forever. In a 6-week study, he had a group of students ride a fan bike for 20 seconds of all-out effort followed by 10 seconds of rest, for 4 minutes straight. The result: The students improved their power endurance by 28 percent. The catch: The students went extremely hard, and, as Tabata himself explained, the workout is "very painful and tiring." He had the students do the workout once each session. I'm going to have you do it 3 times. Get comfortable with discomfort, and improvement is imminent.

DIRECTIONS

You can row, ski, run, or ride a fan bike for this workout. I've also done this on a stair-stepper and an elliptical machine. Work as hard as you possibly can for 20 seconds. Rest for 10 seconds. That's 1 round. Do a total of 8 rounds. Then rest 4 minutes. That makes 1 block. Complete 3 total blocks (which is 24 total rounds).

1. Row, Ski, Run, Fan Bike, Stair-Stepper, or Elliptical: 20 Seconds

2. Rest: 10 Seconds

Blocks: 3, Comprised of 8 Rounds Each (24 Total Rounds)
Time: 24 Minutes

#40

Interval 10
TIME BOMB

Your performance can vary day-to-day based on factors like sleep, stress, and nutrition. So, if you're fully rested and stress-free, you may be able to burn more calories on a 1-minute fan bike test than if you were tired and stressed out. That's why, on some days, I like to ditch specific round or set prescriptions, and just do as many rounds or sets as I can, until my performance drops off. This allows me to get in just the right amount of work, without going overboard (which could ultimately just set me up for injury). This is my favorite workout when I'm not 100 percent in-tune with how I feel, and I just want to get some valuable work in.

DIRECTIONS

Row or ski 100 meters in 20 seconds. Rest for 40 seconds. That's 1 round. Do as many rounds as you can, adding 1 meter to each round, until you blow up and can no longer improve by a meter. So on your second round, you'd need to log at least 101 meters, followed by 102 on your third, and so on. If, on round 17, where your goal would be 118 meters, you only achieve 116, your workout is done. Note: If you can't log 100 meters in 20 seconds, that's completely fine. Start at a distance that requires effort but isn't too hard, and add a meter to that number each round. The best way to do this is by using the intervals/time function on the rower or ski ergometer.

1. Row or Ski: 20 Seconds

2. Rest: 40 Seconds

Rounds: AMRAP, Adding 1 Meter Each Round
Time: 15 to 30 Minutes

#41

Interval 11
FIGHT TEST

The StepMill, or stair-climber, is arguably the most underrated piece of cardio equipment. Go into your average big-box gym, and you rarely see it being used. But it can tax your heart and lungs with the best of them, and there are few training activities more functional than walking up stairs. When I was fighting in the UFC, I'd do this workout to determine if I was fit enough for an upcoming fight. A championship UFC fight is comprised of five 5-minute rounds, each separated by 1 minute of rest. So I'd crank a stair-climber up to its highest level and go for 5 minutes straight, then rest for 1 minute, and then repeat until I'd done 5 total rounds. If I could finish the workout, I knew I was ready to fight.

DIRECTIONS

Climb on a stair-climber set to the highest level you're capable of maintaining for 5 minutes straight. Rest for 1 minute. That's 1 round. Do a total of 5 rounds. If you don't have access to a stair-climber, you could do this workout on stairs at a local high-school stadium, or on a treadmill set to the highest incline.

1. Stair-Climber or Treadmill: 5 Minutes
2. Rest: 1 Minute

Rounds: 5
Time: 30 Minutes

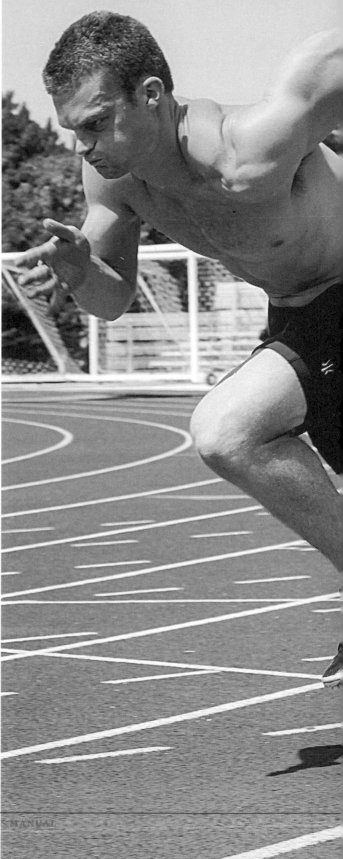

IV: IWT WORKOUTS

In 1987, Pat O'Shea, a competitive weight lifter and exercise scientist at Oregon State University, published a paper in the *National Strength and Conditioning Association Journal* about a new training method he'd spent most of the previous two decades developing. He called it "interval weight training," a high-intensity routine that combines strength and cardio that's done at a blistering pace.

In an IWT (I call it that for short), you do an explosive lift that works your entire body, followed by a fast-paced cardio exercise. You do that for three rounds. That's phase one. In phase two, you select a different strength and cardio exercise, then you do another three rounds.

Over time, I've come to love IWTs. They're my answer for anyone who needs to build strength, endurance, and power in as little time as possible. In fact, I typically do them with a group every Friday. They're hard as hell, and they set the tone for the weekend. Over time, I've developed three types of IWT workouts: general fitness, strength, and endurance.

The workouts listed below are not the be-all, end-all IWT workouts, though. Feel free to make up your own IWTs using the same format, but subbing in different exercises. You can make hundreds of different workouts.

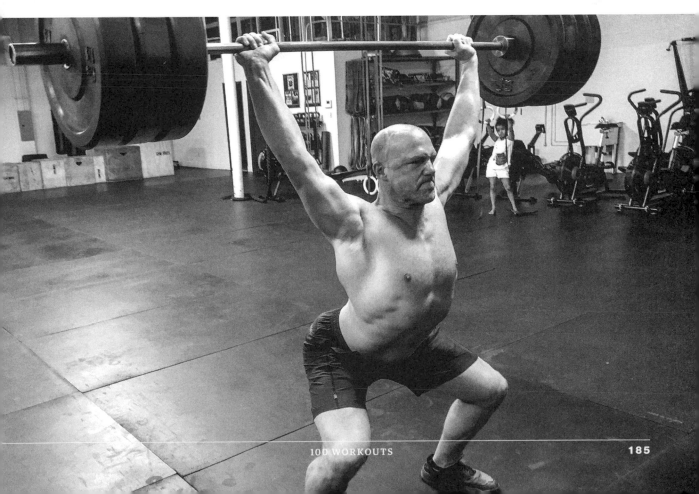

#42

IWT 1
GENERAL

This IWT is great for building all-around fitness—it increases both your strength and endurance. The key is to go hard on the cardio portion: You should be breathing heavy enough that there's no way you could have a conversation. To help people reach that level of exertion, I often give them a distance goal, if they're rowing or skiing. I try to reach 630 meters on the rower or ski ergometer in each 2-minute block but you might start with 550 meters. If you're running or using another piece of equipment, aim for a pace that feels like 90 percent of all-out.

DIRECTIONS

Start with Block 1. Grab a couple dumbbells that weigh around 20 pounds. Do 10 push presses. Immediately ski, row, climb a stair-climber, or run on a treadmill for 2 minutes straight, trying to hit your distance goal. Rest for 2 minutes. That's 1 round. Do a total of 3 rounds. After you complete round 3, rest for 5 minutes. Then, move on to Block 2. Grab a heavy dumbbell or kettlebell and do 10 goblet squats. Immediately row, ski, climb a stair-climber, or run on a treadmill for 2 minutes straight. Rest for 2 minutes. That's 1 round. Do a total of 3 rounds.

BLOCK 1
Push Press: 10 Reps
Ski, Row, Stair-Climb, Run: 2 Minutes
Rest: 2 Minutes

BLOCK 2
Goblet Squat: 10 Reps
Ski, Row, Stair-Climb, Run: 2 Minutes
Rest: 2 Minutes

Rest: 5 Minutes between Blocks
Rounds: 3 of Block 1, then 3 of Block 2
Time: 35 Minutes

#43

IWT 2
STRENGTH

Because you lift heavier weights and focus on going faster over a shorter distance in the cardio exercise, this IWT will hone your strength and power. Like all IWTs, go hard in the cardio portion. In this IWT, I try to reach 475 meters on the rower or ski ergometer in each 90-second block but you might shoot for 425 meters. If you're running or using another piece of equipment, aim for a pace that feels like 95 percent of your all-out effort.

DIRECTIONS

Start with Block 1. Load a barbell with 80 percent of your deadlift 1-rep max. So, if your best deadlift is 350 pounds, the bar should weigh 280. Do 5 deadlifts. Immediately ski, row, climb a stair-climber, or run on a treadmill for 90 seconds straight. Rest for 3 minutes. That's 1 round. Do a total of 3 rounds. After your third round, rest for 5 minutes. Then, move on to Block 2. Load a barbell with 80 percent of your front squat 1-rep max. Do 5 reps. Immediately ski, row, climb a stair-climber, or run on a treadmill for 90 seconds straight. Rest for 3 minutes. That's 1 round. Do a total of 3 rounds.

BLOCK 1
Barbell Deadlift: 5 Reps
Ski, Row, Stair-Climb, Run: 90 Seconds
Rest: 3 Minutes

BLOCK 2
Barbell Front Squat: 5 Reps
Ski, Row, Stair-Climb, Run: 90 Seconds
Rest: 3 Minutes

Rest: 5 Minutes between Blocks
Rounds: 3 of Block 1, then 3 of Block 2
Time: 35 Minutes

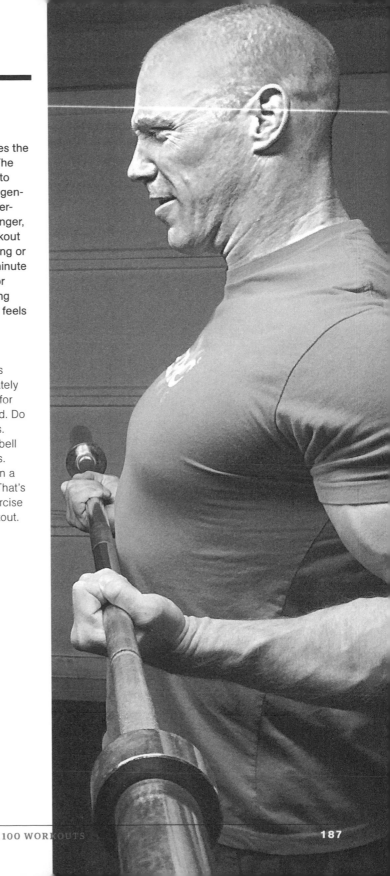

#44

IWT 3
ENDURANCE

This workout is a straight-up kick in the butt. It takes the IWT and turns it into a cardiovascular nightmare. The focus shifts away from strength and goes straight to your lungs. The format and rules are similar to the general IWT, but you do more reps of the weighted exercise, suffer through the cardio portion for much longer, cut your rest down, and do more rounds. This workout sucks, but it'll make you a machine. If you are rowing or on a ski ergometer, aim for 1,100 meters each 4-minute working period. (In case you're wondering, I aim for 1,200 meters when I do it.) If you're running or using another piece of equipment, shoot for a pace that feels like it's about 85 percent of your all-out effort.

DIRECTIONS

Start with Block 1. Grab a couple of light dumbbells (15 pounds is ideal). Do 20 push presses. Immediately ski, row, climb a stair-climber, or run on a treadmill for 4 minutes straight. Rest for 1 minute. That's 1 round. Do a total of 4 rounds. After round 4, rest for 5 minutes. Then, move on to Block 2. Grab a 35-pound dumbbell or a 16-kilogram kettlebell and do 20 goblet squats. Immediately row, ski, climb a stair-climber, or run on a treadmill for 4 minutes straight. Rest for 1 minute. That's 1 round. Do a total of 4 rounds. Finally, pick an exercise from "Finishers" on page 219 to complete the workout.

BLOCK 1
Push Press: 20 Reps
Ski, Row, Stair-Climb, Run: 4 Minutes
Rest: 1 Minute

BLOCK 2
Goblet Squat: 20 reps
Ski, Row, Stair-Climb, Run: 4 Minutes
Rest: 1 Minute

FINISHER
Rest: 5 Minutes between Blocks
Rounds: 4 of Each Block
Time: 35 to 45 Minutes

V: MASS GAIN

Ever since I can remember, I've wanted to be the "Big Guy." When I was a teenager, I wanted to be as muscular as Arnold Schwarzenegger. When I was wrestling, I wanted to compete in the heavyweight division. My career requires me to be big and strong. So, I am. In fact, I consider training to gain muscle my forte.

That said, in *Maximus Body*, you won't put on muscle just to put on muscle. I believe there's no sense in being big without having genuine horsepower to back it up. If you're going to be big, you not only need to be strong, but you also need to be fast, agile, and have stellar endurance. There are only four mass-gain workouts in this book, but they're my absolute, no-question go-to workouts for anyone who wants to add lean mass and be athletic. I've gained an incredible amount of muscle in my life using these simple workouts.

Even if you don't want to gain muscle, these workouts are still absolutely necessary for your fitness. They teach your muscles to deal with stress, and are necessary to rid your body of excess fat—you'll only put on muscle if you're eating enough.

#45

Mass Gain 1
10 BY 10 UPPER

I first started doing 10 by 10 workouts when I was wrestling at the University of Western Ontario in the late 1990s. I needed to gain weight, and by doing these workouts and eating a lot of food, I put on 30 pounds of muscle in just 6 months. Indeed, when it comes to adding muscle, I don't think that there's a better format than 10 sets of 10 reps.

DIRECTIONS
Load a barbell with a weight that you can bench 10 times. Do 10 reps. Then do 10 pullups. If you can't do 10 pullups, do 10 assisted pullups or 10 lat pulldowns. Rest for 2 minutes. That's 1 round. Do a total of 10 rounds. Suggested weights: Beginners, use 135 pounds; intermediates, use 185 pounds; advanced lifters, use 225 pounds.

1. Barbell Bench Press: 10 Reps

2. Pullup: 10 Reps

3. Rest: 2 Minutes

Rounds: 10

#46

Mass Gain 2
10 BY 10 LOWER

I did this workout every single Tuesday of my life for 1 year, and in that time, I went from 217 to a rock-solid 252 pounds. I started out using 135 pounds. When I could complete all 10 sets of 10 reps with that weight, I added 10 pounds and repeated. Eventually, I was doing 10 sets of 10 reps with 315 pounds. Prepare to discover why this is one of the most grueling, soreness-inducing workouts ever. That said, the reward is ginormous, functional wheels. Well worth it, I think.

DIRECTIONS
Load a barbell with a weight that you can back squat 10 times. Do 10 reps. Rest for 2 minutes. That's 1 round. Do a total of 10 rounds. Suggested weights: Beginners, use 135 pounds; intermediates, use 185 pounds; advanced lifters, use 225 pounds.

1. Barbell Back Squat: 10 Reps

2. Rest: 2 Minutes

Rounds: 10

#47

Mass Gain 3
4 BY 15

This is another workout that helped me pack on size. It's done using higher reps than my other mass gain workouts, so it delivers a different training effect, stimulating your muscles to grow. Once you can knock out all your rounds and reps with a given weight, add 10 pounds to the bar next time you do the workout.

DIRECTIONS

Select a barbell exercise: bench press, back squat, front squat, or overhead press. Load the bar with 60 percent of your 1-rep max of the given exercise. So, if your max overhead press is 100 pounds, your bar should weigh 60 pounds. Do 15 reps. Rest for 90 seconds. That's 1 round. Do a total of 4 rounds.

1. Barbell Bench Press, Barbell Back Squat, Barbell Front Squat, or Barbell Overhead Press: 15 Reps

2. Rest: 90 Seconds

Rounds: 4

#48

Mass Gain 4
TICKET TO GAINZVILLE

Silly name, serious results. When I was fighting in the UFC and needed to keep my weight up and maintain my upper-body power, I'd do this barbell circuit. That often surprises people, because many believe that circuits are solely for fat loss. This circuit is different. It's not a race, and the ultimate goal is perfect form. In it, you do a total of 165 reps of three heavy, compound barbell lifts that hit your upper body in different planes of movement. You also do 55 pullups. I've done this workout in just 20 minutes, and afterward felt like I couldn't lift my arms over my head.

DIRECTIONS

Load a barbell. Do 10 reps of the bench press, 10 reps of the pullup, 10 reps of the overhead press, and 10 reps of the bent row. You may need to use two barbells—heavier for the bench, lighter for the overhead press and bent rows. Then, do 9 reps of each exercise, then 8, then 7, and so on, until you do just 1 rep of each. Try to finish the workout quickly, but focus on using perfect form over speed. Rest, as needed, throughout. Select a weight for each exercise that makes it moderately difficult to complete the first 10 reps.

1. Barbell Bench Press

2. Pullup

3. Barbell Overhead Press

4. Barbell Bent Row

Reps: 10, 9, 8, 7, 6, 5, 4, 3, 2, 1 of Each Exercise

VI: NO-GEAR WORKOUTS

People think that you absolutely need equipment to get a good workout. Nonsense. I've had long stints vacationing or traveling for work where I haven't had access to a single weight or machine. I not only didn't let my fitness slide, I actually increased it. All you need to get fit is a floor and an empty space.

You, too, will have times in your life when you have to figure shit out. That's why I created the following no-gear workouts. If you've ever been faced with a situation that keeps you out of the gym, do one of these workouts. You can easily swap one of these in for a weighted workout, and you may even find that they have a greater impact on your fitness.

#49

No-Gear 1
PRISON BURPEES

Imagine that you're in a prison cell, confined by four walls. You have a bed, a sink, a toilet, and no more. When your cell door opens, and it's time to go to the yard, where your safety depends on your fitness. This is the workout you'd do. It's not for the faint of heart, but it has an incredible ability to give you strength, speed, and insane endurance. Do it in 15 minutes or less, and you may be able to claim the title of "the hardest man in the yard."

DIRECTIONS
Stand in one corner of a room—could be in the gym, your living room, garage, wherever. Do 20 burpees. Now run to another corner of the room, and do 19 burpees. Run to another corner, and do 18. Repeat the pattern until you reach 1 burpee. Rest, as needed, throughout.

1. Burpee

Reps: 20, 19, 18, . . . 3, 2, 1
Time: 15 to 25 Minutes

#50

No-Gear 2
SPEED TRIALS

Have an hour and want to boost your fitness across the board without going to a gym? Do this workout. I like it because it's 100-percent running based, but it's not as boring as simply going out for a slow jog for 60 minutes. Switching up speeds not only keeps the workout fresh and motivating but also trains your body to deal with different endurance paces, which boosts your lung power and overall fitness.

DIRECTIONS
Warm up with an easy 10-minute run. Then rest by walking for 3 minutes. Next, do fast intervals: Run fast for 10 seconds at the top of every minute for 10 minutes. Walk for 3 minutes. Do sprint intervals: Sprint for 20 seconds every 2 minutes for 10 minutes. Walk for 3 minutes. Do medium intervals: Run at a medium speed for 1 minute every 3 minutes for 15 minutes. Then, do a 10-minute cooldown run.

1. Warmup Run: 10 Minutes

2. Fast Intervals: 10 Seconds Every Minute, for 10 Minutes

3. Sprint Intervals: 20 Seconds Every 2 Minutes, for 10 Minutes

4. Medium Intervals: 1 Minute Every 3 Minutes, for 15 Minutes

5. Cooldown Run: 10 Minutes

Rest: 3-Minute Walk between Each Exercise
Time: 60 Minutes

#51

No-Gear 3
THE GAUNTLET

In this workout, you do 25 minutes of three classic movements. Prepare to rep out body-weight exercises like squats, pushups, and V-sits; then hold some exercise positions for a certain time; and then finish by taxing your lungs with a run. In the end, you'll be tired from head to toe, but you'll be fitter for it.

DIRECTIONS

Start with a 10-minute warmup run. From there, do the exercises in the order shown below. Do exercises 5A and 5B, 7A and 7B, and 9A and 9B as mini circuits. Do 4 rounds of each. For example, when you get to exercise 5A, do pushups for 30 seconds, and then immediately move on to exercise 5B, in which you hold the bottom position of a pushup for 30 seconds. Without resting, repeat, for a total of 4 rounds. After the fourth round, rest for 2 minutes and then proceed to the next pair of exercises. Use this same procedure for exercises 7A and 7B, and exercises 9A and 9B. Finish with a 20-minute run.

1. Warmup Run: 10 Minutes

2. Wall Squat: 2 Sets, 5 Reps

3. Air Squat: 3 Sets, 20 Reps

4. Jump Squat: 3 Sets, 5 Reps

5A. Pushup: 30 Seconds ——┐
                                   ├ **(4 Rounds)**
5B. Pushup Position Plank: 30 Seconds ┘

6. Rest: 2 Minutes

7A. Air Squat: 30 Seconds ——┐
                               ├ **(4 Rounds)**
7B. Air Squat Hold: 30 Seconds ——┘

8. Rest: 2 Minutes

9A. V-Sit: 30 Seconds ——┐
                        ├ **(4 Rounds)**
9B. V-Sit Hold: 30 Seconds ——┘

10. Cooldown Run: 20 Minutes

Time: 45 Minutes

#52

No-Gear 4
FIRE FIGHT

This is a workout that I teach at every military seminar I lead. It's an incredible routine to have in your back pocket if you're a special forces operator. It doesn't require equipment, and it doesn't take much time—two things most deployed soldiers don't have. The workout improves every aspect of their overall fitness, so they can perform their jobs at the highest level and stay safe. Tackle it with the tenacity of a soldier—it'll be exceedingly difficult, if you're truly willing to go after as many reps as possible.

DIRECTIONS

Do the exercises in the order shown. Complete all the sets of exercise 1, resting, as needed, followed by all the sets of exercise 2 and exercise 3. Then, move on to exercise 4. For this exercise, perform as many reps as you can in 30 seconds, followed by 30 seconds of rest. That's 1 round. Do a total of 4 rounds. On your last round, rest for 2 minutes instead of 30 seconds. Use that same procedure for exercise 6 and exercise 8.

1. Wall Squat: 2 Sets, 5 Reps

2. Air Squat: 3 Sets, 20 Reps

3. Jump Squat: 3 Sets, 5 Reps

4. Burpee: 4 Sets of 30 Seconds Each (Rest for 30 Seconds between Sets)

5. Rest: 2 Minutes

6. Split Jump: 4 Sets of 30 Seconds Each (Rest for 30 Seconds between Sets)

7. Rest: 2 Minutes

8. Frog Hop: 4 Sets of 30 Seconds Each (Rest for 30 Seconds between Sets)

9. Cooldown Run: 10 Minutes

Time: 20 to 25 Minutes

#53

No-Gear 5
TABATA TWO

Time to revisit the dreaded Tabata workout format (see "Interval 9: Tabata Triplets" on page 183) and hammer your entire body. To realize the full effect, do as many reps as you can during each 20-second block of work.

DIRECTIONS

Warm up by doing body-weight movements of your choice for about 10 minutes. Choose exercises such as squats, situps, and pushups. Then, move on to the Tabatas. Do 5 exercises in Tabata format: 20 seconds of hard work followed by 10 seconds of rest, repeated 8 times total. After you finish a given Tabata exercise (4 total minutes), rest for 1 minute, and then move on to the next Tabata exercise. Once you've completed all 5 Tabatas, do a cooldown run for 10 minutes.

1. **Warmup:** 10 Minutes

2. **Air Squat:** 20 Seconds of Work and 10 Seconds of Rest for 8 Rounds

3. **Rest:** 1 Minute

4. **Pushup:** 20 Seconds of Work and 10 Seconds of Rest for 8 Rounds

5. **Rest:** 1 Minute

6. **Leg Raise:** 20 Seconds of Work and 10 Seconds of Rest for 8 Rounds

7. **Rest:** 1 Minute

8. **V-Sit Kickout:** 20 Seconds of Work and 10 Seconds of Rest for 8 Rounds

9. **Rest:** 1 Minute

10. **Burpee:** 20 Seconds of Work and 10 Seconds of Rest for 8 Rounds

11. **Cooldown Run:** 10 Minutes

Time: 44 Minutes

#54

No-Gear 6
HELL STYLE

This workout is the exact same as "No-Gear 5: Tabata Two" at left, except that it's served "Hell-Style." What does that mean? In each Tabata, spend your 10-second "rest" period holding the prescribed "resting position" of the exercise. This workout is psychological torture, and it's about 19 minutes too long. Indeed, it's my go-to for anyone who needs to unf*ck their head.

DIRECTIONS

Warm up with body-weight movements of your choice, such as squats, situps, and pushups. Then, move on to the Tabatas, done "hell style." Do 5 exercises in Tabata hell-style format: 20 seconds of hard work, followed by 10 seconds holding the "resting" position of the given exercise, repeated 8 times total. So, for example, in exercise 2A, you do 20 seconds of air squats. Then, in 2B, you hold the "down" position of a squat (knees bent 90 degrees) for 10 seconds. That's 1 round. Do 8 rounds. Rest for 1 minute (real rest) between each hell-style Tabata.

1. **Warmup:** 10 Minutes

2A. **Air Squat:** 20 Seconds
2B. **Air Squat Hold:** 10 Seconds — (8 Rounds)

3. **Rest:** 1 Minute

4A. **Pushup:** 20 Seconds
4B. **Pushup Position Plank:** 10 Seconds — (8 Rounds)

5. **Rest:** 1 Minute

6A. **Leg Raise:** 20 Seconds
6B. **Leg Raise Hold:** 10 Seconds — (8 Rounds)

7. **Rest:** 1 Minute

8A. **V-Sit Kickout:** 20 Seconds
8B. **V-Sit Hold:** 10 Seconds — (8 Rounds)

9. **Rest:** 1 Minute

10A. **Burpee:** 20 Seconds
10B. **Pushup Position Plank or Air Squat Hold:** 10 Seconds — (8 Rounds)

11. **Cooldown Run:** 10 Minutes

Rounds: 8
Time: 44 Minutes

#55

No Gear 7
30/30 RUNS

This workout is simple and incredibly effective at boosting your speed and performance. I love the format because you can do it anywhere: I've done it on a track, around my neighborhood, or in cities where I've traveled for work. The latter is actually my favorite method. There's no better way to see a new city than by running through it.

DIRECTIONS

Warm up with a slow, 10-minute run. Then, begin the workout: Run fast (but don't sprint) for 30 seconds. Then, run slow for 30 seconds. Repeat that pattern for anywhere from 30 minutes—if you're new to running—to up to 60 minutes, if you're an experienced runner. Finish with 10 minutes of slow running or walking.

1. Warmup Run: 10 Minutes

2A. Fast Run: 30 Seconds

2B. Slow Run: 30 Seconds

3. Cooldown Run: 10 Minutes

Time: 50 to 80 Minutes

#56

No-Gear 8
JENNY'S MATH

This workout is named after my friend Jenny. A few years ago, she traveled to Alaska to do some archaeological work. She had zero access to gear, but told me she wanted one workout that she could do at a football field that was across the street from where she was staying. I sent her this workout, which has a whole hell of a lot of bear crawls (I thought it appropriate, being that she was in Alaska). Here's the kicker: When I sent it, she e-mailed me back to ask how many yards are in a meter. I told her that 1 meter is equal to 2 yards, a bold-faced lie that meant she was doing twice the distance of bear crawling that I had actually prescribed. She thought I was telling the truth, and two things happened: One, she became insanely fit, and two, she hasn't trusted me since.

DIRECTIONS

Do the exercises in the order shown. Start with a lower-body warmup (exercises 1 and 2), resting, as needed. Then, move on to exercises 3A and 3B. Do 20 split jumps followed immediately by 50 meters of the bear crawl. That's 1 round. Do a total of 5 rounds, rest for 2 minutes after, and then move on to exercises 5A and 5B. Follow the same procedure for exercises 5A and 5B, but only do 4 rounds. Rest. For exercises 7A and 7B, do 3 rounds. Finish with the cooldown run.

1. Air Squat: 3 Sets, 20 Reps

2. Jump Squat: 3 Sets, 5 Reps

3A. Split Jump: 20 Reps ⎤
3B. Bear Crawl: 50 Meters ⎦ **(5 Rounds)**

4. Rest: 2 Minutes

5A. Frog Hop: 20 Reps ⎤
5B. Bear Crawl: 40 Meters ⎦ **(4 Rounds)**

6. Rest: 2 Minutes

7A. Burpee: 20 Reps ⎤
7B. Bear Crawl: 30 Meters ⎦ **(3 Rounds)**

8. Cooldown Run: 10 Minutes

Time: 45 Minutes

#57

No-Gear 9
THE JACKED KANGAROO

Jumping is an incredible exercise. You see it in nearly every sport, and even if you don't play sports, it builds raw power. That not only transfers to every exercise but also helps you reach your desired physique. This workout requires something to jump onto, but it doesn't have to be a box. I've used a patio, rocks, tree stumps—anything that's sturdy and won't fall over. The only limit is your imagination. Judging by how jacked some kangaroos are (no kidding: Google that sh*t), jumping does wonders.

DIRECTIONS

Do the exercises in the order shown. Complete all of the sets in exercise 1, then move on to exercise 2 and exercise 3. Rest, as needed, between sets of all three exercises. Perform exercise 4A and 4B as a mini circuit: Do one set of the box jump followed immediately by one set of the pushup position plank, and then rest for 30 seconds. That's 1 round. Do a total of 4 rounds. Note: For the box jump, try to jump onto a sturdy surface that's about 20 inches high. For Exercise 5, do 100 pushups as fast as you can, resting, as needed, then rest for 1 minute.

1. Air Squat: 3 Sets, 20 Reps

2. Jump Squat: 3 Sets, 10 Reps

3. Tuck Jump: 4 Sets, 5 Reps

4A. Box Jump: 25 Reps

4B. Pushup Position Plank: 1 Minute (4 Rounds)

4C. Rest: 30 Seconds

5. Pushup: 100 Reps

6. Cooldown

Time: 30 Minutes

#58

No-Gear 10
IT'S HARDER THAT WAY

You know what's harder than running? Running up a hill. Know what's harder than running up a hill? Jumping up a hill. The upshot is that you'll build more power in your lower body, and your heart rate will go through the roof, helping improve your endurance.

DIRECTIONS

Start with a warmup comprised of body-weight exercises of your choice. Then do frog hops up a hill or a flight of stairs for 30 seconds. Rest for 30 seconds. That's 1 round. Do a total of 6 rounds, and then rest for 3 minutes. That's 1 block. Complete a total of 3 blocks.

Now move on to exercise 4. Do 10 seconds of pushups, and then rest for 20 seconds. That's 1 round. Do a total of 15 rounds. Finally, finish with the cooldown run.

1. Body-Weight Warmup: 5 Minutes

2. Frog Hop Uphill: 30 Seconds of Work Followed by 30 Seconds of Rest for 6 Rounds

3. Rest: 3 Minutes

4. Pushup: 10 Seconds of Work Followed by 20 Seconds of Rest for 15 Rounds

5. Cooldown Run: 5 Minutes

Blocks: 3

Time: 45 Minutes

#59

No-Gear 11
THE STEEPER THE HILL . . .

. . . the greater the challenge. Which is why, for this workout, I want you to find the steepest hill in your town. Then, you're going to sprint up it, so you become stronger and faster. Don't have a hill, or can't go outside? Set a treadmill to the highest incline and go. Enjoy.

DIRECTION

Warm up with an easy 10-minute run. Then do a 10-minute progressive speed run: Start slow and continuously gain speed so you end in a fast run. Recover completely. Then sprint uphill—or on a treadmill set to the highest incline—for 1 minute straight. Rest for 4 minutes, taking the time to walk or stretch. That's 1 round. Do a total of 5 rounds. Afterward, jog or walk for 15 to 30 minutes to cool down.

1. Warmup Run: 10 Minutes

2. Progressive Speed Run: 10 Minutes

3. Uphill Sprint: 1 Minute of Work Followed by 1 Minute of Rest for 5 Rounds

4. Cooldown Jog or Walk: 15 to 30 Minutes

Time: 40 to 60 Minutes

#60

No-Gear 12
28 MINUTES

When I lead fitness seminars, each workout I give is designed to teach people a lesson that they can incorporate into their daily training. The lesson of this workout: Excuses are bullshit. You can do this workout anywhere in less than half an hour.

DIRECTIONS

Do the exercises in the order shown. Perform each exercise for 30 seconds, followed by 30 seconds of rest. That's 1 round. Complete a total of 4 rounds of the prescribed exercise, rest for 2 minutes, and then move on to the next exercise. So, you do 4 rounds of the frog hop, rest for 2 minutes, followed by 4 rounds of the split jump. Repeat the pattern until you finish the last round of squats.

1. Frog Hop: 30 Seconds of Work Followed by 30 Seconds of Rest for 4 Rounds

2. Rest: 2 Minutes

3. Split Jump: 30 Seconds of Work Followed by 30 Seconds of Rest for 4 Rounds

4. Rest: 2 Minutes

5. Burpee: 30 Seconds of Work Followed by 30 Seconds of Rest for 4 Rounds

6. Rest: 2 Minutes

7. Pushup: 30 Seconds of Work Followed by 30 Seconds of Rest for 4 Rounds

8. Rest: 2 Minutes

9. Air Squat: 30 Seconds of Work Followed by 30 Seconds of Air Squat Hold

Time: 28 Minutes

#61

No-Gear 13
10 TO 1

This is a great workout to do while watching TV. You pack in a ton of quality work—55 reps of 5 different exercises—and perform the entire workout in one spot. I'll do this at home while catching up on my favorite series on Netflix, or when I'm stuck in a hotel room. I've listed my go-to exercises below, but you can sub in your own.

DIRECTIONS

Do the exercises in the order shown. Start with 10 reps of the pushup, then do 10 air squats, 10 situps, 10 burpees, and 10 lunges (1 on each leg counts as 1 rep). Then repeat, but do 9 reps of each movement. Continue this pattern, doing 1 less repetition each round all the way down to 1 rep.

1. Pushup

2. Air Squat

3. Situp

4. Burpee

5. Lunge

Reps: 10, 9, 8, 7, 6, 5, 4, 3, 2, 1
Time: 20 Minutes

#62

No-Gear 14
200 IN 20

This workout tasks you with doing 200 total reps, and trains your entire body in just 20 minutes. It's short, simple, and brutal, just the way I like my workouts. It's easy to remember, too, so many of my athletes keep it in their heads as an option for when they find 20 minutes to train. Don't cheat your form, but try to finish as fast as you possibly can.

DIRECTIONS

Do 10 pushups, 10 situps, and 10 air squats. That's 1 round. Complete a total of 20 rounds. Try to finish in less than 20 minutes.

1. Pushup: 10 Reps

2. Situp: 10 Reps

3. Air Squat: 10 Reps

Rounds: 20
Time: 15 to 30 Minutes

#63

No-Gear 15
GO LONGER

In this workout, you'll be tested to do a set amount of pushups, lunges, and air squats every minute, on the minute for as long as you possibly can. The first 10 minutes will feel easy. But soon, fatigue will creep in. Once you reach minute 20—if you reach minute 20—you'll be hanging on for dear life. Your goal: 30 minutes. If you hit this target, you'll have accumulated 150 pushups, 300 lunges, and 450 squats, which is more than most people do in a week.

DIRECTIONS

Set a stopwatch or timer, ideally one that beeps every minute (there are free smartphone apps that do this). Every minute, on the minute, do 5 pushups, 10 lunges (each leg counts as 1 lunge), and 15 air squats. The workout is done when you can't meet your prescribed reps in any minute. Go as long as you can.

1. Pushup: 5 Reps
2. Lunge: 10 Reps
3. Air Squat: 15 Reps

Rounds: AMRAP
Time: 10 to 30 Minutes

#64

No-Gear 16
A MARRIAGE MADE IN HELL

Running and burpees: A marriage made in the darkest depths of hell. Indeed, two of the hardest tests I know are the 1.5-mile test and the 100-burpee test. This workout wraps both of those god-awful tests together into one workout. But look on the bright side, you only have to do 75 burpees instead of 100.

DIRECTIONS

Run a half-mile, then do 25 burpees. That's 1 round. Do 3 rounds as fast as you can.

1. Run: 0.5 Mile
2. Burpee: 25 Reps

Rounds: 3
Time: 15 to 20 Minutes

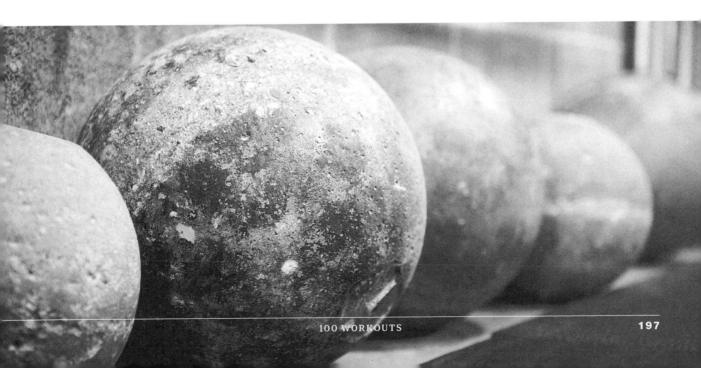

VII. BIRTHDAY WORKOUTS

As I age, I want to improve, not decline. My goal is to be as fit at 40 as I was at 20. I want to be as fit at 50 as I was at 30. That's why, every year on my birthday, I wake up and celebrate by immediately doing one of the savage workouts in this section. It's not just a test. It's also a reminder that I'm becoming fitter with age, and that I still have the ability to improve no matter what year my birth certificate says I was born.

The "Birthday Workouts" have actually become something of a phenomenon in my community. People now ask me to give them the gift of a birthday workout. It's almost a rite of passage.

Here are my two favorites. They're hard enough that you'll be glad you only have one birthday a year.

#65

Birthday 1
HAPPY F%^KING BIRTHDAY

Instead of asking for a birthday workout, a few of the over-age-35 people who train with me guard the date of their birth like it's a precious diamond. They don't want me to know their age or DOB because they know I'll give them this age-based workout, and they don't want to undergo the suffering. News flash: I always find out the age and birthdate of everyone who trains with me, and I'm okay with my friends hating me on their birthday.

DIRECTIONS

Take your age. That's how many air squats and lunges you do. That's 1 round. What was your age again? That's how many rounds you do. So, for example, if you're turning 35 years old, you'll do 35 air squats and 35 lunges, 35 times. That's 2,450 total reps. Happy birthday!

1. Air Squat: Your Age in Reps

2. Lunge: Your Age in Reps

Rounds: Your Age
Time: Depends on Your Age

#66

Birthday 2
BIRTHDAY GAINZ

The bench press is my favorite exercise. That's why, if I really like you, I'll let you bench press for your birthday workout. (That can be a very good or a very bad thing.) For my 37th birthday, I did 37 sets of 37 reps using 135 pounds. It worked out to 1,369 reps.

DIRECTIONS

Take your age. That's how many reps and sets of bench press you do. So, for example, if you're 30, you'll do 30 sets of 30 reps. Choose your weight wisely.

1. Bench Press: Your Age in Reps

Sets: Your Age
Time: Depends on Your Age

VIII. STRENGTH AND POWER WORKOUTS

Strength and power are two of the most important physical attributes you can have. Strength is the max force that you can produce, while power is how fast you can apply that force. Think of the former as the ability to grind out a rep with a very heavy weight, while the latter would be more akin to the ability to jump extremely high.

The two characteristics are key, because they tend to stick with you for the long haul. If you work your way up to a massive deadlift or an eye-popping vertical leap, you can possess these two skills for longer, compared to cardiovascular fitness, which you constantly have to train to maintain.

For example, I've seen people who haven't deadlifted for a month pull a personal record, and guys who haven't jumped in months still hop onto a 50-inch box. On the other hand, it's horrifying what happens when a person who hasn't done cardio in a month takes a 100-burpee test.

These workouts will help you develop a very high level of strength and power, two skills that are critical in any goal, whether that's elite fitness, building muscle, pulling a huge deadlift, running a marathon, or just avoiding injury when you do activities you love.

In these workouts, strict attention to good form is critical. There's an inherent risk to lifting heavy weights—the heavier the weight, the bigger the risk. Mitigate that risk by stressing form over the number on the bar.

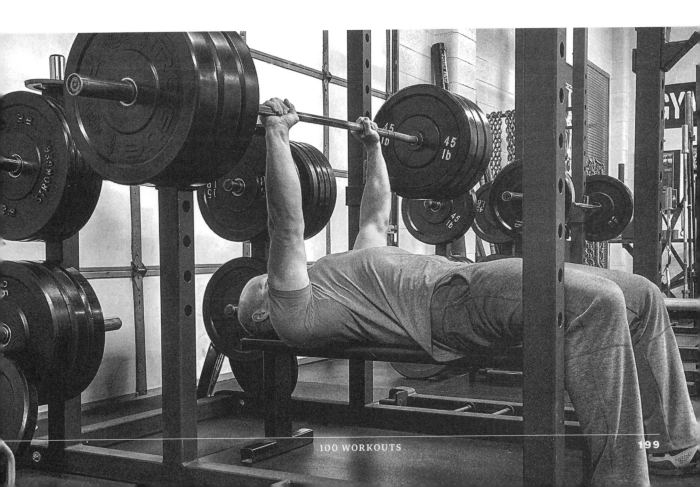

#67

Strength and Power 1
5 BY 2 AT 80

When it comes to lifting heavy, you don't always have to push the envelope. Sometimes, you might want to just maintain your strength—for instance, because you're running a marathon or cutting weight—rather than build it. In that case, I have people do this workout. It should also leave you feeling energized.

DIRECTIONS

Choose just one exercise from the list below. Load a barbell with a weight that's equivalent to 80 percent of your 1-rep maximum (see "Max Tests" on page 159). If your 1-rep max deadlift is 350 pounds, you'd lift a bar weighing 280. Do 2 reps with perfect form. Rest for 3 minutes. That's 1 round. Do a total of 5 rounds.

Barbell Bench Press

Barbell Overhead Press

Barbell Front Squat

Barbell Back Squat

Barbell Overhead Squat

Barbell Deadlift

Reps: 2
Rest: 3 Minutes after 2 Reps
Rounds: 5
Time: 20 Minutes

#68

Strength and Power 2
6 BY 2 AT 85

This workout is a strength-builder. At first glance, it looks similar to "Strength and Power 1: 5 by 2 at 80" at left. But, notice that you use a heavier weight, and you perform an additional set. This workout is actually my go-to when I want to build strength over time.

DIRECTIONS

Choose one exercise from the list below. Load a barbell with a weight that's equivalent to 85 percent of your 1-rep maximum (see "Max Tests" on page 159). If your 1-rep max deadlift is 350 pounds, you'd lift a bar weighing slightly less than 300 pounds. Do 2 reps with perfect form. Rest for 3 minutes. That's 1 round. Do a total of 6 rounds.

Barbell Bench Press

Barbell Overhead Press

Barbell Front Squat

Barbell Back Squat

Barbell Overhead Squat

Barbell Deadlift

Reps: 2
Rest: 3 Minutes after 2 Reps
Rounds: 6
Time: 25 Minutes

#69

Strength and Power 3
4 BY 4 AT 80

This is, by far, one of the best workouts I know of to not only build strength but also to build strength endurance. Doing 4 reps of a weight that's equal to 80 percent of your 1-rep max is taxing. Because of that, the workout is riskier than the following two workouts (you're more likely to get injured on reps 3 and 4), but it also has incredible payouts. That last set will feel like a grind, but it results in rapid improvements in strength.

DIRECTIONS

Choose an exercise from the list below. Load a barbell with a weight that's equivalent to 80 percent of your 1-rep maximum (see "Max Tests" on page 159). So, if your 1-rep max deadlift is 350 pounds, you'd lift a bar weighing 280. Do 4 reps with perfect form. Rest for 4 minutes. That's 1 round. Do a total of 4 rounds.

Barbell Bench Press
Barbell Overhead Press
Barbell Front Squat
Barbell Back Squat
Barbell Overhead Squat
Barbell Deadlift

Reps: 4
Rest: 4 Minutes after 4 Reps
Rounds: 4
Time: 20 Minutes

#70

Strength and Power 4
6 BY 1 AT 90

There's nothing more empowering than loading a bar with an ungodly amount of weight and doing 1 difficult rep. That's exactly what you do in this workout, and I consider it a real man-maker. It delivers the greatest benefits in terms of raw strength. This is the workout you should be doing if you're training to hit a new 1-rep max.

DIRECTIONS

Choose an exercise from the list below. Load a barbell with a weight that's equivalent to 90 percent of your 1-rep maximum (see "Max Tests" on page 159). So, for example, if your 1-rep max deadlift is 350 pounds, you'd lift a bar weighing 315. Do 1 rep with perfect form. Rest for 5 minutes. That's 1 round. Do 6 rounds.

Barbell Bench Press
Barbell Overhead Press
Barbell Front Squat
Barbell Back Squat
Barbell Overhead Squat
Barbell Deadlift

Reps: 1
Rest: 5 Minutes after 1 Rep
Rounds: 6
Time: 30 Minutes

#71

Strength and Power 5
ADD 5

Doing exercises to failure is critical for building size and strength. In this workout, you're not going to follow any weight percentages. You're just going to start with a weight of 75 pounds, do the 3 exercises listed, add 5 pounds to the bar, and repeat. Once you hit failure in one of the exercises (likely exercise 1), ditch the first exercise, and continue to do the other two, continuing to add 5 pounds to the bar each set. Once you fail at one of the remaining two exercises, keep adding weight but only do the remaining exercise. Once you fail, your upper body will be completely gassed, and you'll have set yourself up for strength and size.

DIRECTIONS

Load a bar so it weighs 75 pounds. Do 2 barbell overhead presses, 2 barbell push presses, and 2 barbell jerks. Add 5 pounds to the bar, and repeat (your rest occurs when you're loading the bar). Continue the pattern—adding 5 pounds to the bar each set—until you can no longer do the 2 barbell overhead presses. Without changing the weight on the bar, do 2 barbell push presses and 2 barbell jerks, continuing to add 5 pounds to the bar every set. Once you can't do 2 barbell push presses, do just 2 jerks, adding 5 pounds to the bar every set. Once you can't do 2 jerks, you're done.

1. Barbell Overhead Press: 2 Reps

2. Barbell Push Press: 2 Reps

3. Barbell Jerk: 2 Reps

Sets: As Many as Possible, Adding 5 Pounds to the Bar Each Set
Time: 15 to 45 Minutes

#72

Strength and Power 6
100-REP CHALLENGE

This is another workout inspired by the great strength coach, Dan John. It asks you to perform just 1 rep—100 times. You can almost think of it as a 1-rep, 100-set workout. Daunting, right? Indeed, this challenge is as much psychological as it is physical. Focus on making each rep absolutely perfect. Prepare to see great improvements to your form and strength.

DIRECTIONS

Pick an exercise from the list. Load a bar with 50 percent of your 1-rep max (see "Max Tests" on page 159). If you can barbell back squat 400 pounds, you'll use 200 pounds for this. Do 1 rep. Re-rack the bar. Rest for 15 seconds. That's 1 set. Do 100 rounds.

Barbell Bench Press
Barbell Overhead Press
Barbell Front Squat
Barbell Back Squat
Barbell Overhead Squat
Barbell Deadlift

Reps: 1
Rest: 15 Seconds between Each Rep
Rounds: 100
Time: 30 Minutes

#73

Strength and Power 7
SPEED KILLS

In sports, power and speed kill. Run faster and jump higher than your competition, and you have a clear advantage. I do this workout with all the NBA and NFL athletes I work with. Jump squats at 30 percent of your body weight elicit an incredible power response. And adding a difficult power movement to that only drives home the explosion. If you want to build quickness and hop like a pro, do this workout once a week for 8 weeks.

DIRECTIONS

Load a barbell so it weighs 30 percent of your body weight. If you weigh 200 pounds, for example, your bar would weigh 60 pounds. Do 2 reps of barbell jump squats, jumping as high as you can each rep. Re-rack the bar and do one of the power movements listed. Rest for 2 minutes. That's 1 round. Do 8 rounds.

1. Barbell Jump Squat: 2 Reps
2. Box Jump (3 Reps), Sled Sprint (25 Yards), Sprint (40 Yards), or Sprint Row (10 Seconds)

Rest: 2 Minutes between Rounds
Rounds: 8
Time: 25 Minutes

#74

Strength and Power 8
POWER PLAY

The combination of deadlifting and jumping is a tremendous tool to build your power and explosiveness. Doing a heavy lower-body lift followed by an explosive move elicits a phenomenon called postactivation potentiation, which allows you to recruit more motor neurons and become stronger and more powerful. This workout, in particular, is my personal go-to for when I want to work on my own strength and power, and I teach it at many of the fitness seminars I lead.

DIRECTIONS

Load a barbell so it weighs 80 percent of your 1-rep max (see "Max Tests" on page 159) for deadlifts. If your max is 500 pounds, the bar would weigh 400 pounds. Do 2 reps of the deadlift. Once you're done, immediately do 5 broad jumps, trying to jump as far as possible. Don't rush them. Take about 10 seconds between each jump to properly set up. Rest for 4 minutes. That's 1 round. Do 5 rounds.

1. Barbell Deadlift: 2 Reps
2. Broad Jump: 5 Reps

Rest: 4 Minutes between Rounds
Rounds: 5
Time: 30 Minutes

#75

Strength and Power 9
ROCKET BOOSTERS

In this workout, you grind through the heavy barbell front squat, then explode in the box jumps. This elicits the phenomenon of postactivation potentiation (see "Strength and Power 8: Power Play" on page 203), which helps you realize greater gains in strength and power. Don't rush through this workout. Make sure that your front squat reps are perfect and that your box jumps are done with as much power as possible. If you do the box jumps correctly, you will feel like you are attached to a rocket.

DIRECTIONS

Load a barbell so it weighs 80 percent of your 1-rep max (see "Max Tests" on page 159) for front squats. If your max is 200 pounds, the bar would weigh 160 pounds. Do 3 reps of the front squat, making sure to move the weight cleanly (it'll still feel like a grind). Immediately do 5 box jumps, trying to jump as high as possible. Don't rush them. Take about 10 seconds between each jump to properly set up. Rest for 3 minutes. That's 1 round. Do 5 rounds.

1. Barbell Front Squat: 3 Reps
2. Box Jump: 5 Reps

Rest: 3 Minutes between Rounds
Rounds: 5
Time: 30 Minutes

#76

Strength and Power 10
ALL OUT

In the introduction to the first section of this book, I talked about the all-out minute fan bike test. It's one of the most brutal tests of fitness, mental fortitude, and willpower I know.

It also happens to be an incredible way to develop power across a longer span—1 full minute as opposed to the second it takes to lift a weight or complete a jump. That's important for any sport where you need to be powerful for a handful of seconds: in a fight, sprinting in soccer, battling for a rebound. If your goal is just to look good, the test is an incredible way to pack in intense work, which raises your metabolism for hours. Track your calorie burn or distance, and try to improve each time that you do this workout.

DIRECTIONS

Ride a fan bike, ski ergometer, rower, or run as hard as you possibly can for 1 stupid minute straight. One round is enough: If you don't feel absolutely wrecked at the end of this, you didn't go hard enough.

1. Fan Bike, Ski, Row, Run: 1 Minute

Time: 1 Minute

IX: CHALLENGES

I believe that humans were built to be tested. Without trials, we would have no sense of where our capabilities lie, or whether we're improving. In the gym, I use tests to determine the unseen by-products of exercise, like psychological resilience, willpower, and heart and soul—I can test whether the deep chemical changed I talked about in Section I: Psychology (see page 1) has occurred.

The mind is primary, and there are so many more benefits to training than just looking good naked. Training makes your mind stronger and can affect everything from your marriage to your job to your ability to be a parent.

Challenges are what bring these changes to the surface. They're what push you to the precipice, helping you discover who you really are. These are what forge your spirit.

The goal with these challenges is to try your absolute hardest, always in an attempt at improvement.

#77

Challenge 1
2K ROW

When people do circuits for time, they can cheat form and cut corners. But, when it comes to the rowing machine, it is just you and the computer: You can't cheat, and there are no shortcuts, just objective feedback staring you in the face. That's why I consider the 2,000-meter row the ultimate test of grit. It tests your power endurance, of course, but also the power of your spirit. I ask that the people I train finish it in 7 minutes or less. That's a long time—long enough to find yourself or long enough to talk yourself into quitting.

DIRECTIONS
Set a rowing machine's computer for 2,000 meters. Row the distance as fast as you can. If you don't want to quit at the halfway point, you're not going hard enough. Pro tip: Set the rower's damper (the dial on its fan) somewhere between 4 and 8.

1. Row: 2,000 Meters

Goal Time: 7 Minutes or Less
Time: 6 to 8 Minutes

#78

Challenge 2
100 BURPEES FOR TIME

You can do this workout anywhere, anytime. You don't need gear, and you don't need a gym. Do it in a park, in your basement, at the office, wherever. All you need is a will to suffer and a desire to find out what you're made of. Your goal is to finish in 6 minutes or less. The rule: Each burpee must be of quality form. Your chest must touch the ground, and you must jump a minimum of 6 inches at the top. I'd rather see you take 7 minutes to do 100 perfect burpees than 5 minutes to do 100 half-assed ones.

DIRECTIONS
Start a stopwatch. Do 100 burpees as fast as you possibly can.

1. Burpee: 100 Reps

Goal Time: 6 Minutes or Less
Time: 6 to 10 Minutes

79

Challenge 3
CAN'T VS. WON'T

This workout tests your will to succeed more than your fitness. When you do it, you're going to face what I call "the moment." That's the point during a workout where your brain tells you to shut it down and quit. You can believe it, quit, and stay the same, or, you can persevere, pushing onward to find an improved version of yourself. When you're finished, ask yourself, *Was it my mind or body that decided when the workout ended?*

DIRECTIONS

Set a rowing machine's computer's interval setting to 30 seconds of work and 90 seconds of rest. Row 140 meters and no more. Take your 90 seconds of rest. That's 1 round. Next round, row 141 meters and no more, followed by 90 seconds of rest. Continue to add 1 meter to each round until you "can't" or "won't" go any farther.

1. Row: 30 Seconds

2. Rest: 90 Seconds

Rounds: 30, Adding 1 Meter Each Round
Time: 30 to 90 Minutes

80

Challenge 4
2K SKIERG

This workout is very similar to the "Challenge 1: 2K Row" on page 205, except you use a ski ergometer. You may not be familiar with the ski ergometer, unless you go to a CrossFit gym, but it might be my favorite piece of equipment. Unlike the rower or a fan bike, you stand, so you carry your own weight throughout, which has a better cardiovascular effect. In this test, aim for a time that's equivalent to your fastest 2K row time. That's harder to attain for most people, but we don't lower standards. We only raise them.

DIRECTIONS

Set a ski ergometer's computer for 2,000 meters. Ski the distance as fast as you can. If you don't want to quit at the halfway point, you're not going hard enough.

1. Ski Ergometer: 2,000 Meters

Goal Time: 7 Minutes or Less
Time: 7 to 8 Minutes

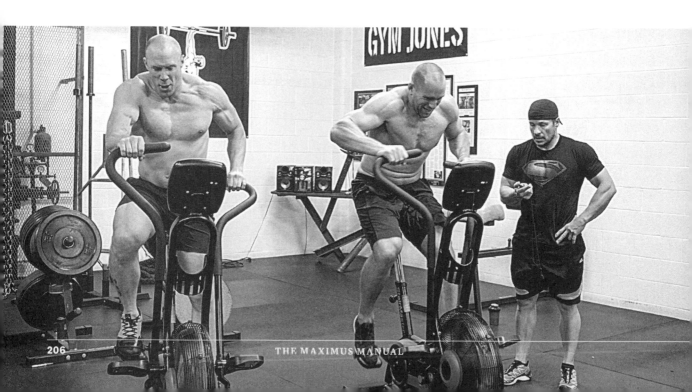

#81

Challenge 5
THE TRIATHLON

The three cardio machines I use most are the rower, ski ergometer, and the fan bike. One day, a guy I train named Doug came up with a twisted idea: "Why don't we combine all three of them?" No one in the gym has forgiven him since.

This is the hardest workout you can do in 5 minutes or less. It's a three-part, all-out sprint to the finish that I've never seen a person walk away from normally. Pro tip for logging a faster time: Go hard but slightly pace yourself on the ski ergometer, go completely balls-to-the-wall on the bike, and simply hang on and give everything you have left on the row. My best time is 3:58. Even the memory of it hurts.

DIRECTIONS

Set a stopwatch. Ski for 500 meters. Ride a fan bike until you hit 50 calories. Row 500 meters. Try to finish each as fast as you can.

1. Ski: 500 Meters
2. Fan Bike: 50 Calories
3. Row: 500 Meters

Goal Time: 5 Minutes or Less
Time: 4 to 7 Minutes

#82

Challenge 6
THE TREADMILL DRILL

In addition to the "Interval 11: Fight Test" on page 184, I also used this test to gauge if I was ready for the grind of five, 5-minute rounds in an MMA ring. I learned it from legendary fighter Bas Rutten. When I could complete this test, my conditioning was where it needed to be, and if I couldn't finish, I'd work on my endurance until I could. The workout is a true grind, but when you can do 6 rounds, you're in pretty damn good shape.

DIRECTIONS

To warm up, run for 8 minutes on a treadmill set to a speed of 7.3 miles an hour with no incline. Rest for 2 minutes. As you rest, set the treadmill to its max incline—15 is ideal—and a speed of 6.3 miles an hour. To begin the rounds, run on the treadmill for 45 seconds. Rest for 30 seconds. That's 1 round. Try to log 6 rounds. By the way, holding yourself up on the treadmill's railings is not allowed.

1. Treadmill Run Warmup: 8 Minutes
2. Rest: 2 Minutes
3. Uphill Treadmill Run: 45 Seconds, followed by 30 Seconds of Rest for 6 Rounds

Time: 20 Minutes

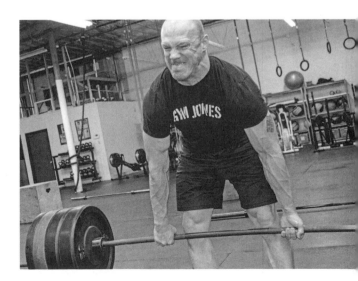

#83

Challenge 7
2-MILE TIME TRIAL

When I wrestled at the University of Western Ontario, our coach started the season with a test that showed him whether or not we'd each trained in the off-season. He'd take us down to the track and make us run 2 miles as fast as possible. Eight laps around a track is a long way to run if you've let your cardio slip, a fact I learned the hard way my second season. That off-season, I'd lifted a lot of weights and become strong, but I'd completely neglected cardio, because I didn't like it. My terrible experience and finishing time taught me one of the most important lessons in fitness: When you have a goal, you can't take a break from doing things you don't like. Progress requires discomfort.

DIRECTIONS

Run 2 miles as fast as you can. That's 8 laps around a track. You can also use a GPS watch, or run on a treadmill.

1. Run: 2 Miles

Goal Time: 12 Minutes or Less
Time: 10 to 16 Minutes

#84

Challenge 8
Z-PRESS TEST

This exercise is an overhead barbell press that you perform while sitting on the floor. By taking your lower body out of the equation, you're forced to rely solely on your core and upper body for strength. This test is a great way to tell if your upper body and core strength need improvement, because you can cheat other upper-body lifts by engaging your legs. Pro tip: Break your reps into mini sets. If you go to fatigue during your first set, you'll burn out early.

DIRECTIONS

Grab an unloaded barbell and sit up straight, on the floor, with your legs in front of you. Set a timer for 10 minutes. Do as many reps as you can.

1. Barbell Z-Press: 10 Minutes

Goal Reps: 200 or More
Time: 10 Minutes

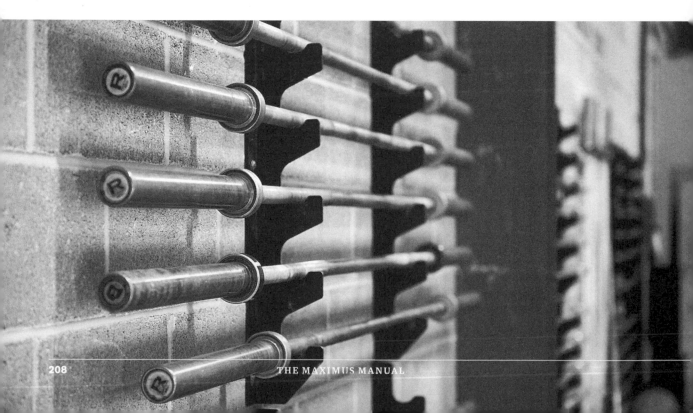

#85

Challenge 9
AIR SQUAT TEST

Simple but brutal: Do as many reps of air squats as you can in 10 minutes. Because there's no weight involved, you're forced to focus completely on your range of motion and form every rep. This test also serves as a great workout for athletes who have to hammer their legs nonstop for a set amount of time, such as downhill skiers, Nordic skiers, 5K runners, and more. There isn't much strategy to this test—just go all-out.

DIRECTIONS

Set a timer for 10 minutes. Using good form, do as many air squats as you can.

1. Air Squat

Goal Reps: 450 or More
Time: 10 Minutes

#86

Challenge 10
MDL AT 225

I learned this test from the Ranger Athlete Warrior Program, an Army Ranger training program. In all the work I've done with the rangers, I enjoy this test the most. It challenges just how much you can pick up from the ground in a given time, something that's incredibly applicable not only to fighting in a war zone but also to working around the house, playing with their kids, and more. In it, complete as many unbroken 225-pound deadlifts as you can.

DIRECTIONS

Load a barbell so it weighs 225 pounds. If you can't deadlift that much, it's okay to go lighter and work up to 225 pounds over time. Spot up to the bar, and deadlift it as many times as you possibly can in a row. Use good form. If you feel your form slipping, ditch the bar instead of grinding out ugly reps, which can set you up for injury.

1. Barbell Deadlift

Goal Reps: 25 or More
Time: 3 Minutes

#87

Challenge 11
MAX PULLUPS

Seeing how many pullups you can do in a row is one of the most tried-and-true upper-body strength tests. It's a great indication of your power-to-weight ratio, and the biggest, strongest guy doesn't always perform best. In fact, you have an advantage if you're smaller. This test is used by many military selections. Shoot for the standard set by the Marine Corps: 15 reps.

DIRECTIONS

Hang from a pullup bar and do as many pullups as you can. You can change your grips midway through, but your feet can't touch the ground. You're done if your feet touch the ground or you can't do any more.

1. Pullup

Goal Reps: 15 or More
Time: 3 Minutes

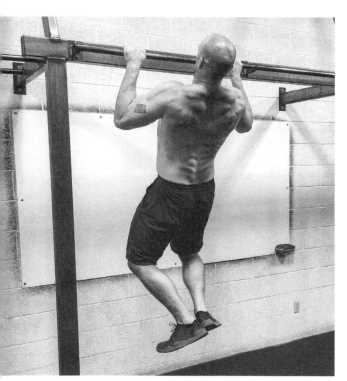

#88

Challenge 12
MAX PUSHUPS

The pushup test is perhaps the most classic strength test. You probably did it in gym class. I've taken hundreds of pushup tests in my life, but my favorite comes from the Ontario Police College in Canada. Lots of my fellow cadets and I went into that test thinking that we were going to crush it. But, because of its strict design that forced us to use proper form and not cheat reps, many of us logged far less reps than we hoped. But our pushups were correct, so our lower numbers were actually more indicative of our true ability.

DIRECTIONS

Start by lying on your stomach, your hands on the floor under your shoulders, your feet together. Keep your body perfectly straight and do a pushup, taking 1 second to push yourself up, and 1 second to lower yourself. Make sure that your chin touches the mat at the bottom of every rep. If your form deviates or you spend more than 2 seconds in the "up" or "down" position, you're done.

1. Pushup

Goal Reps: 45 or More
Time: 5 minutes

#89

Challenge 13
MAX CURLUPS

This is the ultimate abs endurance test. You're forced to do reps slowly so you can't use momentum to log shoddy reps. Back when I was a cop in Toronto, we had to take this test annually as part of our police physicals. My abs would burn for a week afterward, but it was a good burn.

DIRECTIONS

Take this test with a metronome (there are many metronome smartphone apps available for free). Set the metronome for 50 beats per minute. Do curlups at a pace of 25 per minute. So, for example, on the first beep go "up," and on the second beep go "down." Do as many reps as you can until you fail.

1. Curlup

Goals Reps: 75 or More
Time: 3 Minutes

#90

Challenge 14
SACRAMENT

Not only is this upper-body strength test featured in the NFL Combine, it's also the official test of the "Church of Bobby Maximus." You know my goal is to be the "Big Guy," and there's really nothing that packs more mass onto your upper body than doing a lot of bench reps with a heavy weight.

DIRECTIONS

Load a barbell so it weighs 225 pounds. If you cannot bench that weight, that's no problem. Use a bar that weighs equal to your body weight. If you weigh 150 pounds, for example, use a bar that weighs 150 pounds (or lighter, if need be). Make sure that the bar touches your chest at the bottom, and your arms lock out at the top. Do as many reps as possible.

1. Barbell Bench Press

Goals Reps: AMRAP
Time: 2 Minutes

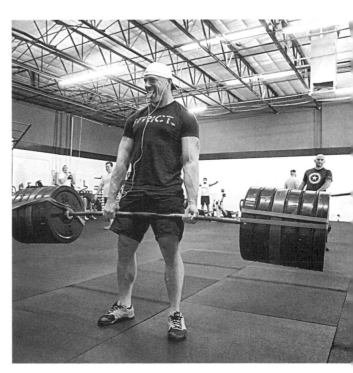

91

Challenge 15
20 MINUTES OF MAYHEM

Short on time but need an absolute ass-kicking workout? Here's your ticket. Pair three barbell exercises with three body-weight moves, and go for broke for 20 minutes straight. The only strategy is to simply keep doing reps. Once you finish one move, go directly to the next. If you can think clearly, try to count your reps. If all you did was this workout 5 days a week, you'd be on your way to insane fitness.

DIRECTIONS

Load barbells with appropriate weight for barbell back squats, bench presses, and push presses (shoot for a weight that you can do 15 reps of for each). Set a timer for 20 minutes and begin. Do as many reps of the exercises listed below as you can until the timer goes off. One rep of any exercise is 1 point. Try to score as many points as possible. Pro tip: Go back and forth between the upper- and lower-body exercises.

1. Barbell Back Squat

2. Barbell Bench Press

3. Body-Weight Lunge

4. Burpee

5. Barbell Push Press

6. Pushup

Goal Reps/Points: 400 or More
Time: 20 Minutes

92

Challenge 16
100-REP BENCH OR SQUAT CHALLENGE

I do this workout anytime I need to break through a plateau—it shocks your system with weight and intensity, eliciting progress. It's rather simple: Load a barbell and do 100 reps of the back squat or bench press as fast as you can. The key is to follow my weight recommendations. Notice in the directions I have very specific weights laid out. People often ask me to adjust the weight so it's more "fair" for their body weights. Here's what I tell them: "Shit in the real world weighs what shit weighs. You can't push a button to magically alter the mass of something so it's more 'fair' for your body weight." But if you work toward these weights, I promise that you'll see progress across the board.

DIRECTIONS

Pick either the barbell bench press or the barbell back squat. The first time you take this test, load a bar so it weighs 135 pounds. Do 100 reps of the exercise as fast as you possibly can. If you can finish all your reps in 10 minutes or less, use 185 pounds next time. Once you can do all the reps in 10 minutes with 185 pounds, move up to 225 pounds. Once you can do all the reps with 225 pounds, you're officially part of the "Big Guy Club."

1. Barbell Back Squat or Barbell Bench Press

Goal Reps: 100 or More
Time: 10 Minutes

#93

Challenge 17
30-MINUTE BENCH OR SQUAT CHALLENGE

This is similar to "Challenge 16: 100-Rep Bench or Squat Challenge" at left, except it's three times as long. You're going to load a barbell and see how many reps of the barbell back squat or bench press you can do in 30 minutes. I recommend using a bar that weighs 225 pounds, and, at the gym, I'm the king of the bench press. My best in this test is 272 reps. Tommy Hackenbruck, who took second place in the CrossFit Games in 2009, is the undisputed champion of the squat version of this test. I once saw him do 269 reps. P.S. If you can beat Tommy, please video it and send it to me so I can inform him that he's been dethroned.

DIRECTIONS

Pick either the barbell back squat or bench press, then load the bar with a weight you can do 10 reps of. If you want to try the standard I use at The Church of Bobby Maximus, the bar should weigh 225 pounds. Set a timer for 30 minutes. Do as many reps as you can until the timer goes off.

1. Barbell Back Squat or Barbell Bench Press

Goal Reps: 200 or More
Time: 30 Minutes

#94

Challenge 18
100 BURPEE PULLUPS

And you thought that 100 normal burpees for time was bad. This takes the test to a whole new level by adding a pullup to each rep. This test becomes very nightmarish very fast. But, it also works your strength and endurance, hits every muscle in your body, and will make you a machine—so it's well worth it, in my opinion.

DIRECTIONS

Do 100 burpee pullups as fast as you possibly can. Pro tip: Pace yourself. Don't rocket out of the gate. Find a pace that you can sustain throughout.

1. Burpee Pullup

Goal Reps: 100 or more
Time: 10 Minutes

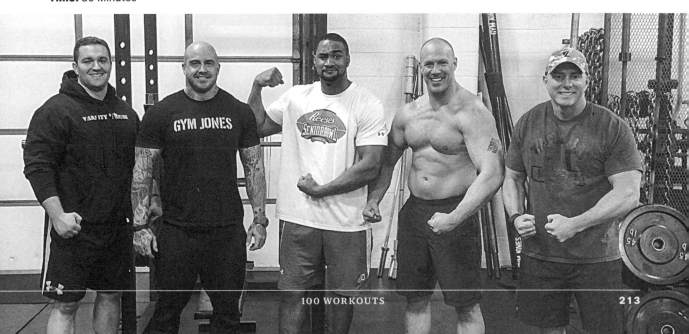

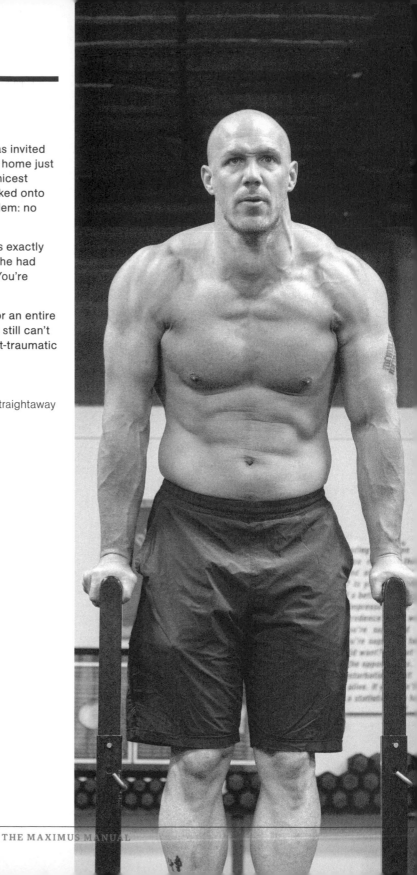

95

Challenge 19
1-MILE LUNGE

I was teaching a seminar in England and was invited to stay at my good friend George's country home just outside of London. His home is one of the nicest places I have ever seen—I felt like I had walked onto the set of a movie—but there was one problem: no gym.

The solution: A road near his home that was exactly 1 mile long. I casually asked him one day if he had ever lunged it. He looked at me and said, "You're bloody insane."

Challenge accepted. Together we lunged for an entire mile without resting. To this day, he says he still can't drive on it without feeling some kind of post-traumatic stress disorder.

DIRECTIONS

Lunge for 1 mile straight. Can be done on a straightaway or on a track (4 total laps).

1. Lunge

Distance: 1 Mile
Time: 75 Minutes

X: TIME TRIALS

These cardiovascular efforts develop your ability to breathe, to recover quickly, and to lose body fat. They're also extremely effective tests of your willpower and general fitness.

Don't take these workouts lightly—everyone wants to lift heavy weights because it feels good, but these workouts are where champions are made. Don't believe me? I did these workouts leading up to every one of my successful fights, and I had Hack's Pack do them regularly before their two CrossFit Games team championships.

#96

Time Trial 1
1.5-MILE RUN

When I was a police officer, you had to pass this time trial, or you were politely asked to hand in your badge and gun. We had to take the test to even receive our badge and gun in the first place. I remember wanting to log a perfect score on the physical fitness exam—which also included bench press, 40-yard dash, leg press, and pullup tests—and this was my greatest impediment. For a perfect score, I'd have to finish in under 9 minutes. I trained my ass off, and, at a weight of 225, logged a time of 8:52.

DIRECTIONS
Run 1.5 miles as fast as you can. That's 6 laps around a standard track. Pro tip: Don't go too hard your first lap, or you'll blow up on lap 6.

1. Run: 1.5 Miles

Goal Time: 9 Minutes or Less
Time: 7 to 15 Minutes

#97

Time Trial 2
5K RUN

Five kilometers is a brutal running distance. For most people, 2 miles is doable. It's hard, but doable. The addition of a mile changes things. It's short enough that you have to run very hard, but long enough that you can't just go all out, or you'll blow up late. In an odd conundrum, it takes pacing so you don't go too hard, but not so much pacing that you don't go hard enough. I used this test with Hack's Pack, CrossFit Games team champions, regularly, and I'm rather sure they still hate me for it.

DIRECTIONS
Run 5 kilometers as fast as you can.

1. Run: 5 Kilometers

Goal Time: 22 Minutes or Less
Time: 15 to 30 Minutes

#98

Time Trial 3
MAKE WEIGHT

I was eating a massive steak dinner with my good friend Johnny when my phone rang. A Las Vegas number displayed across the screen. It was Joe Silva, the head matchmaker for the UFC. He had a fight for me in the 205-pound weight class, and wanted to know if I was interested. At the time, I weighed exactly 242 pounds. I slid my steak dinner away from me, told Joe I'd take the fight, and went for my first 10K run that night. My body naturally wants to sit around 240 pounds. To stay light, I need to run. So, I started running a 10K five times a week, in the morning on an empty stomach, and, sure enough, I made weight at the fight. This run is a slower pace than the 1.5-mile and 2K and 3K runs. But the key is to keep moving and push yourself, which is why I consider it more of a psychological challenge than a physical one.

DIRECTIONS

Run 10 kilometers as fast as you can.

1. Run: 10 Kilometers

Goal Time: 50 Minutes or Less
Time: 30 to 65 Minutes

#99

Time Trial 4
MAX METERS IN 30

This half-hour test tells me just how hard you're willing to push yourself for a relatively short period of time. It's a mental crucible, but it can have a remarkable effect on your spirit and fitness—if, and only if, you're willing go hard. My personal best is 8,700 meters. Try to log 8,000.

DIRECTIONS

Set a rower or ski ergometer's computer for 30 minutes. Begin, trying to log as many meters as possible.

1. Row or Ski

Goal Distance: 8,000 Meters
Time: 30 Minutes

#100

Time Trial 5
MAX METERS IN 60

This is my favorite way to test a person's cardiovascular fitness. It's also a great indicator of someone's mental strength. Sixty minutes is a hell of a long time to sit on a rower and stare at its small computer screen. Weak-minded people break down. Do you slow down even when you don't need to? Do you get up and take a drink even though you don't need to? Do you accept a lower score because you don't like a bit of discomfort? Prepare to find out.

DIRECTIONS

Set a rower's computer for 60 minutes. Begin, trying to log as many meters as possible. If you don't have a rower, run as far as you can in 1 hour.

1. Row

Goal Distance: 15,400 Meters
Time: 60 Minutes

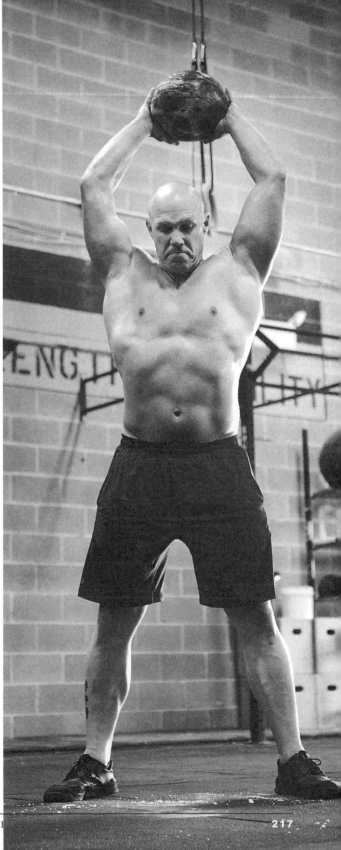

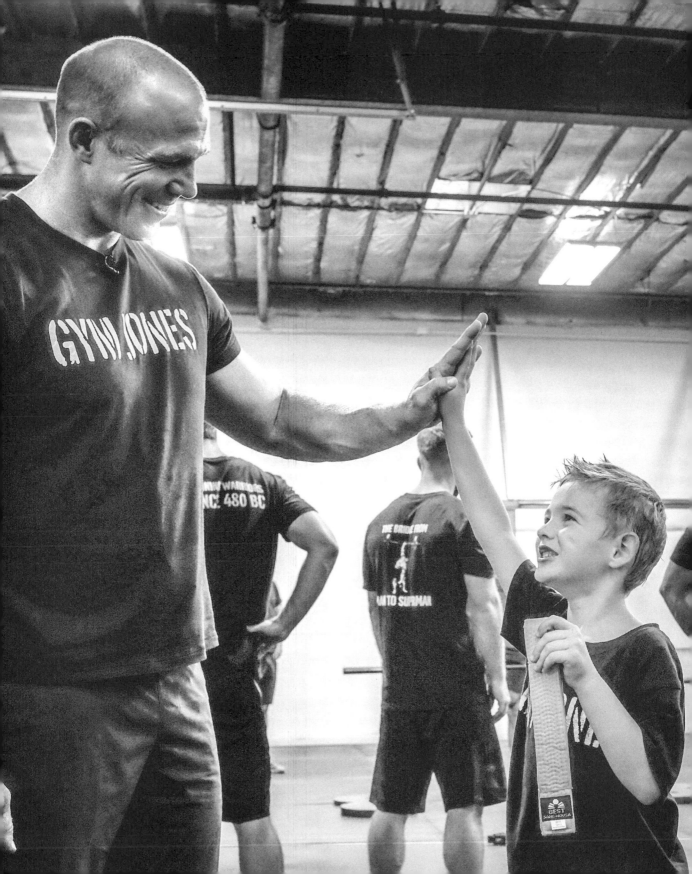

25

FINISHERS

The more fit you become, the more you need extra work in order to keep improving. That's why we often do "finishers" after the primary workout of the day.

Sometimes, finishers are designed to correct imbalances, work on your exercise technique, or injury-proof your body. Other times, the finisher is meant to be a final ass-kicker of the day in order to improve your general fitness.

I like to cycle through finishers, and try to improve each time I do any of them. Below are my 10 favorite finishers, all of which take less than 10 minutes.

Finisher 1
500-METER ROW

This finisher boosts your power endurance. Do it as quickly as possible, and aim to finish in less than 1:30. Done right, you'll feel like you've done enough work for the day.

DIRECTIONS

Set a rower's computer to 500 meters. Row, trying to complete the distance as quickly as possible.

1. Row: 500 Meters

Goal Time: 1:30

Finisher 2
1K ROW

Half the distance of the 2K row, it's not as mentally and physically arduous, but it allows you to really push the pace for an extended period of time. Your goal: 3:30.

DIRECTIONS

Set a rower's computer to 1,000 meters. Row, trying to complete the distance as quickly as possible.

1. Row: 1,000 Meters

Goal Time: 3:30

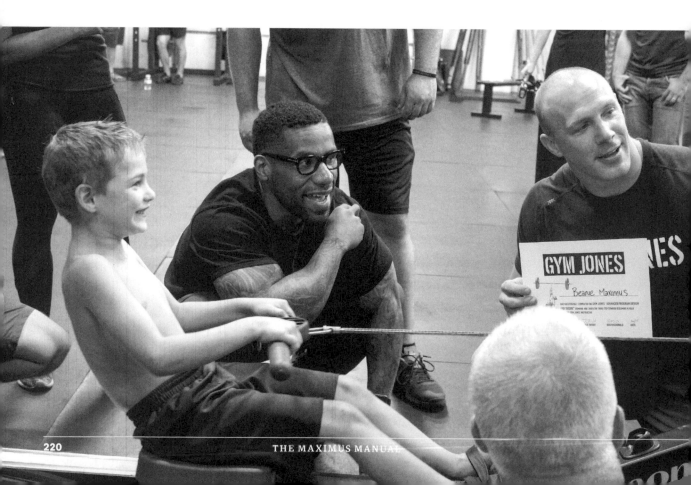

Finisher 3
300FY

A few years ago, an incredible number of people were doing the "300" workout and posting their times online. There were some times that were just so incredibly fast, they were impossible. It was pretty evident that these people were using terrible form, half-reps, etc. Because of that, 300FY was devised. It's done on a fan bike for calories. You can't cheat form or do half-reps; all you can give is incredible effort. If you don't get 300 calories in 10 minutes, I'm sure you can guess what FY stands for.

DIRECTIONS

Ride a fan bike for 10 minutes, trying to burn as many calories as possible. Your goal: 300. If you don't have a fan bike, aim for 3,000 meters in 10 minutes on a rower.

1. Fan Bike (300 Calories) or Rower (3,000 Meters)

Time: 10 Minutes

Finisher 4
1-MILER

How bad could just 1 mile be? It all comes down to how much you are willing to suffer. Shoot for 6 minutes or less.

DIRECTIONS

Run a mile as quickly as you can.

1. Run: 1 Mile

Goal Time: 6 Minutes or Less

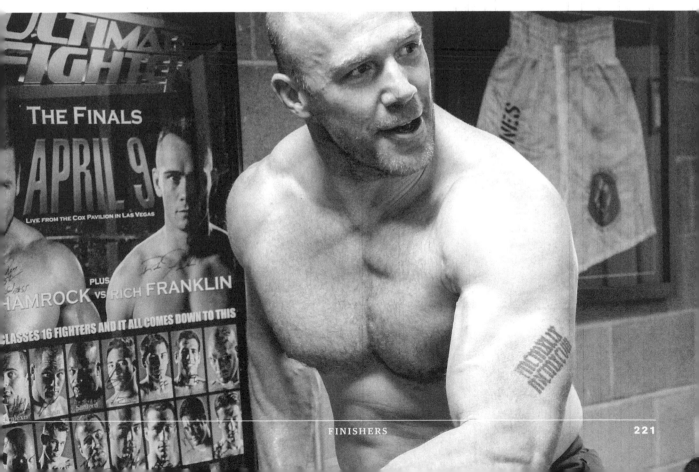

Finisher 5
QUICK AND DIRTY

This is my favorite short interval. I do it after most strength workouts. It has a unique ability to not only reset my body after the hard work but also to improve my overall fitness.

DIRECTIONS

Row, ski, or run hard for 20 seconds. Rest for 40 seconds. That's 1 round. Do 4 rounds. That's 1 block. Rest for 2 minutes, then repeat, this time with one of the remaining exercises.

Block 1. Row, Ski, Run: 20 Seconds of Work, 40 Seconds of Rest for 4 Rounds

Rest: 2 Minutes

Block 2. Row, Ski, Run: 20 Seconds of Work, 40 Seconds of Rest for 4 Rounds

Blocks: 2 (8 Total Rounds)
Time: 10 Minutes

Finisher 6
PULLUP LADDER

Most people are weak in the pullup. That's because they just don't do enough of them. The pullup is an exercise you need to practice to improve in—there are no shortcuts. This finisher packs 105 reps into 10 minutes.

DIRECTIONS

Do 1 pullup. Rest for 5 to 10 seconds. Do 2 pullups. Rest for 5 to 10 seconds. Do 3 pullups, then 4, and so on, until you reach 6 reps. That's one ladder. Do 5 total for 105 reps.

1. Pullups: 1, 2, 3, 4, 5, 6 Reps
Ladders: 5

Time: 10 Minutes

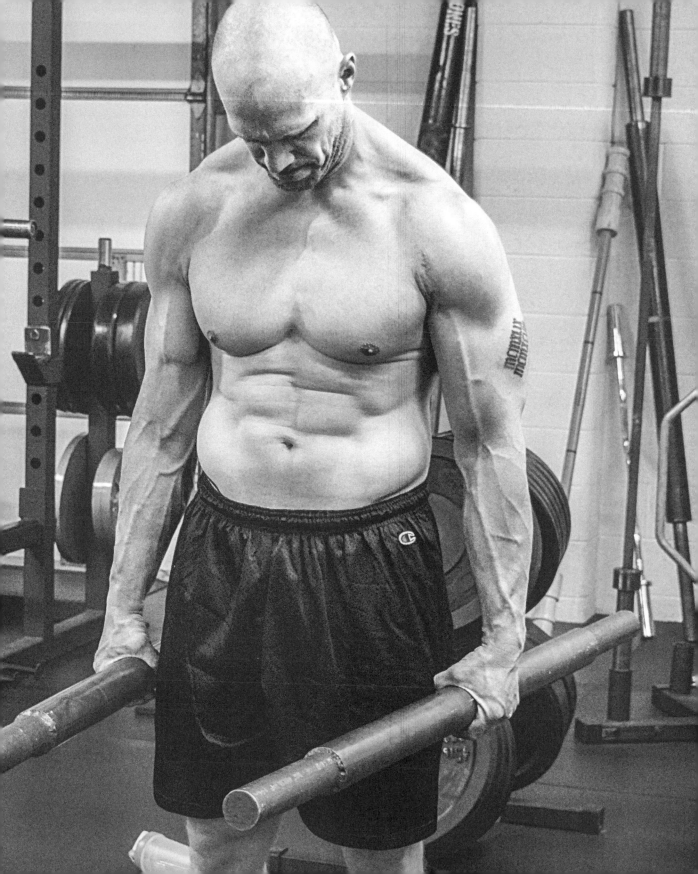

Finisher 7
5-MINUTE PLANK

A strong core makes you stronger in every single lift, and also helps you prevent injury. The way to bolster your midsection? Spend a lot of time in the plank position. It can be that simple.

DIRECTIONS

Assume a pushup plank position and hold it for 5 minutes, squeezing your abs throughout.

1. Pushup Position Plank

Time: 5 Minutes

Finisher 8
PUSHUP MAXIMUS

This is one of the very first pushup workouts I ever did, and I immediately fell in love. It only takes about 3 minutes, but once you can do 10 unbroken reps every set, you have a strong upper body.

DIRECTIONS

Do 10 pushups. Rest for 10 seconds. That's 1 round. Do 10 rounds.

1. Pushup: 10 Reps
2. Rest: 10 Seconds

Rounds: 10
Time: 3 to 4 Minutes

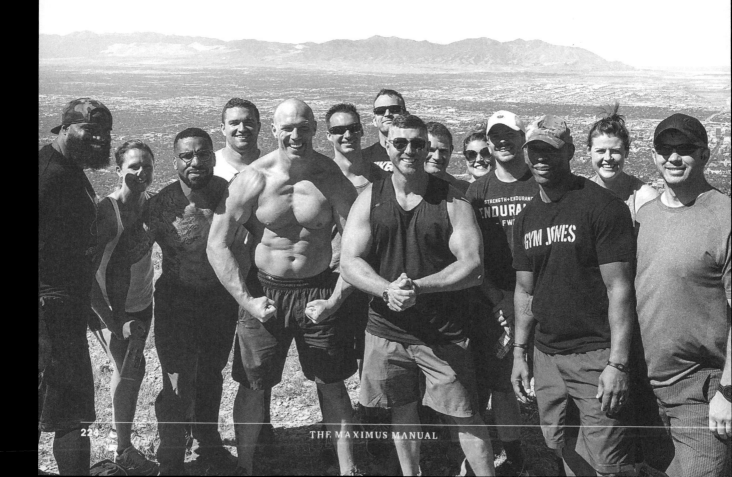

Finisher 9
5QOR

QR stands for "quality reps." I included that in the name because I really want to stress it. This finisher isn't about finishing fast. I want you to stress form over speed, so you can see better injury-prevention, strength, and muscle-building benefits.

DIRECTIONS

At the top of each minute, do 5 pushups, 5 dips, and 5 pullups. Continue the pattern for 10 minutes.

1. Pushup: 5 Reps

2. Dip: 5 Reps

3. Pullup: 5 Reps

Time: 10 Minutes

Finisher 10
THE BEST FOR LAST

Remember the all-out minute from the intro section (see page 2)? Now it's time to see what you're made of. Go as hard as you possibly can. If you're not destroyed afterward, you didn't go hard enough.

DIRECTIONS

Go all out for 1 minute on a rower, fan bike, or running.

1. Row, Fan Bike, or Run: 1 Minute

Time: 1 Minute

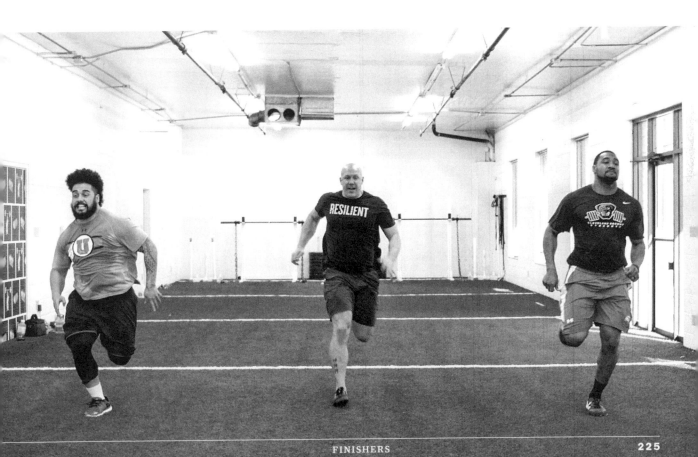

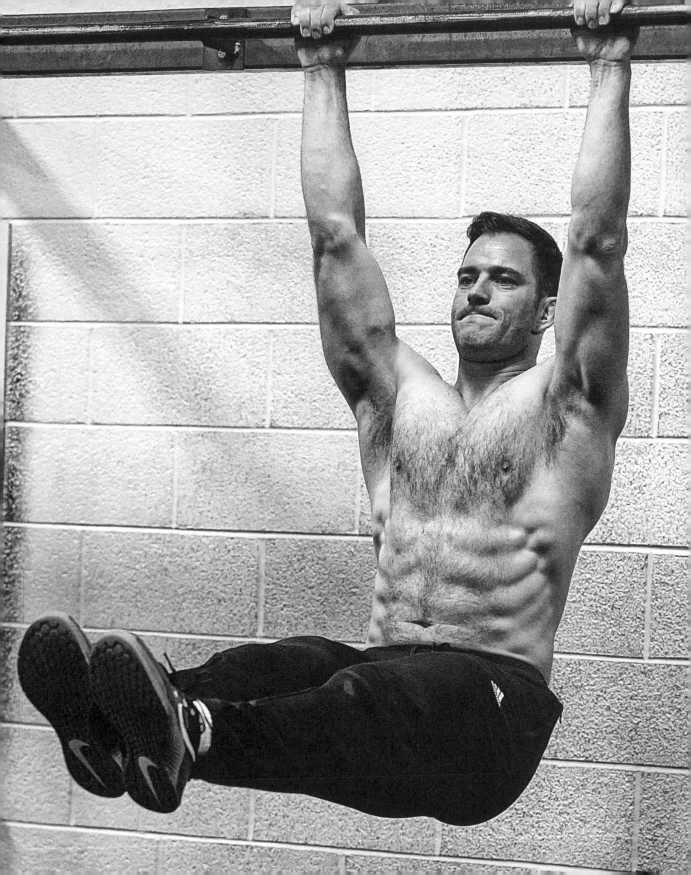

26

RECOVERY WORKOUTS

After a hard workout, your body goes into recovery mode, rebuilding your muscle and resetting your system. That's how you improve your fitness. But during the period between hard workouts, doing nothing will delay that process. (Read more in Chapter 18.) The following recovery workouts are done at low intensity, but they increase blood flow to your muscle and increase your fitness skills, helping you reach your goal faster.

There are two types of recovery workouts: weighted and cardiovascular. Weighted recovery workouts correct imbalances, improve your exercise technique, and build specific fitness attributes. Cardiovascular recovery workouts increase blood flow, flush your muscles, burn calories and fat, and build overall cardiovascular fitness.

Recovery 1
60 AT 70

In this session, maintain a heart rate that's equivalent to about 70 percent of your max heart rate for a full hour. For a 40-year-old, it's around 130 beats per minute. Since you probably don't wear a heart rate monitor all the time, just work at a pace where you're sweating but can have a conversation the entire time. Remember, this is a recovery workout. Don't go too hard.

DIRECTIONS

Pick a cardio exercise from the list and perform it for 60 minutes at an easy pace. If you wear a heart rate monitor, try to stay at 70 percent of your max heart rate. If you don't, don't go so fast that you can't carry on a full conversation.

Row

Run

Cycle

Fan Bike

Stair-Climb

Swim

Time: 60 Minutes

Recovery 2
EASY INTERVALS

I love a good, hellish interval workout. These are not those types of intervals. I do this workout, frankly, because some days I find "60 at 70" to be a bit boring. To break up the monotony of just sitting for 60 minutes on a machine, I go about three-quarters of my usual interval speed, and don't work more than 20 seconds on any one interval. I also take a nice 40-second rest between each interval. You shouldn't feel exhausted after this.

DIRECTIONS

Start with a 10-minute general warmup done at an easy pace. Then pick a cardio activity, and do it for 20 seconds at about 75 percent of your top speed. Rest for 40 seconds. That's 1 round. Do 30 rounds, then finish with a 10-minute cardio cooldown at an easy pace.

1. Easy-Pace Row, Run, Bike, Stair-Climb: 10 Minutes

2A. Row, Run, Cycle, Fan Bike, Ski, Stair-Climb: 20 Seconds

2B. Rest: 40 Seconds (30 Rounds)

3. Easy-Pace Row, Run, Bike, Stair-Climb: 10 Minutes

Rounds: 30 of 2A and 2B
Time: 50 Minutes

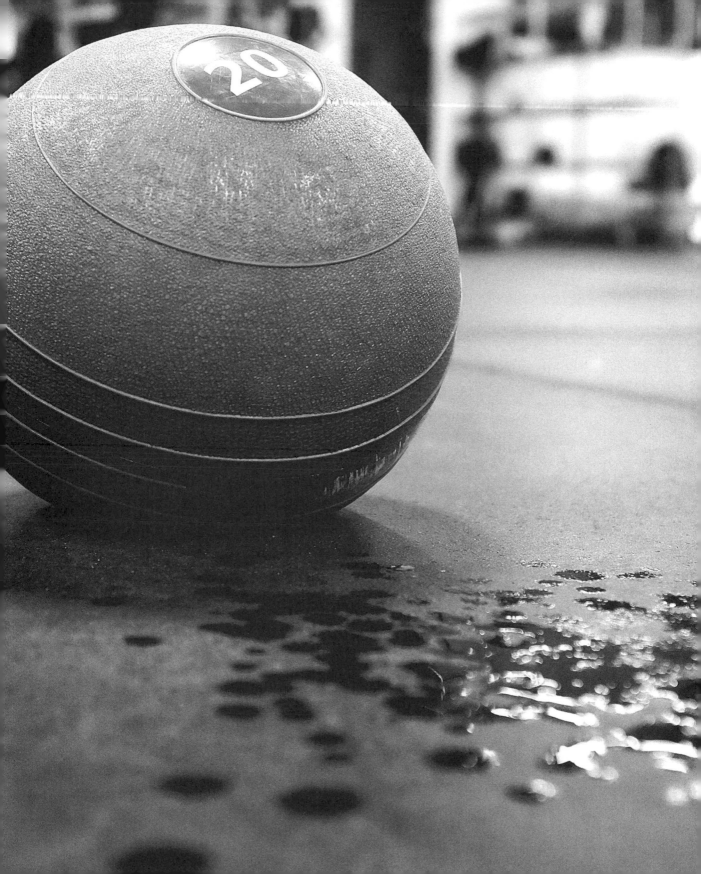

Recovery 3
FARTLEK FUN

Fartlek is Swedish for "speed play." It's an unstructured interval run, where you go from easy to moderate to hard efforts at random. It's also fun to do with friends by playing games like follow the leader. There's a huge mental benefit from this training due to its unpredictability—ditch your watch, your distance goals, and all your other numbers and just go out, have fun, and keep it free flowing.

DIRECTIONS

Run for 60 minutes. Spend most of your time at an easy pace, but randomly throw in hard and moderately paced intervals. You might, for example, jog slowly down the sidewalk then sprint from a street sign to a tree, then jog slowly again.

1. Run

Time: 60 Minutes

Recovery 4
UPPER-BODY RECOVERY

The pullup, dip, and pushup is my favorite exercise combination. Together, they'll build you a strong, powerful upper body that's capable of handling anything the world throws at you. If this was a hard workout, I'd do the exercises for time. But because this is a recovery workout, do the reps at an easy pace, and focus on form. You want to leave the gym fresh, not crushed.

DIRECTIONS

Do the pushups, pullups, and dips in any order you want. Do 50 reps of each exercise. Don't push too hard or rush things. You might, for example, do 5 pushups, 5 pullups, and 5 dips, repeated at a slow pace.

1. Pushup: 50 Reps

2. Pullup: 50 Reps

3. Dip: 50 Reps

Time: 10 Minutes

Recovery 5
100 TURKISH GETUPS

The Turkish getup delivers a whole hell of a lot of benefits: It balances your core, stabilizes and mobilizes your shoulders, builds your overhead work capacity, and also elevates your heart rate. In this workout, you do 100 reps with a light weight, which fixes a lot of mobility and stability issues in your body. Remember, the goal isn't speed. Do each rep slow and controlled, at the gym or at home. It'll take you around 30 minutes, and it will feel monotonous, which is exactly why it also doubles as a great psychological test.

DIRECTION

Grab a dumbbell weighing 15 to 20 pounds. Do 100 Turkish getups, doing 50 on each side.

1. Turkish Getup: 100 Reps

Time: 30 Minutes

Recovery 6
FIX YOUR FORM

When someone comes to me and says they hurt their back, the culprit is usually the deadlift. It's a technically demanding lift that requires diligent attention to form. One bad movement can easily tweak your back. This recovery workout hones your deadlift form so that you're less likely to slip into poor form on your heavy deadlift days.

DIRECTIONS

Load a barbell with a weight that's equivalent to 30 percent of your 1-rep max (don't know that number? Just use 95 to 135 pounds). So, for example, if your max deadlift is 400 pounds, you'd use 120 pounds. Do 20 slow, controlled reps. Don't speed through these—focusing on form is key. That's 1 set. Do 3 sets, then prop the weights on a weight plate, and repeat. Finish with 5 minutes of pushup position planks.

1. Barbell Deadlift: 3 Sets, 20 Reps
2. Deadlift on Plates: 3 Sets, 20 Reps
3. Pushup Position Plank: 5 Minutes

Time: 15 Minutes

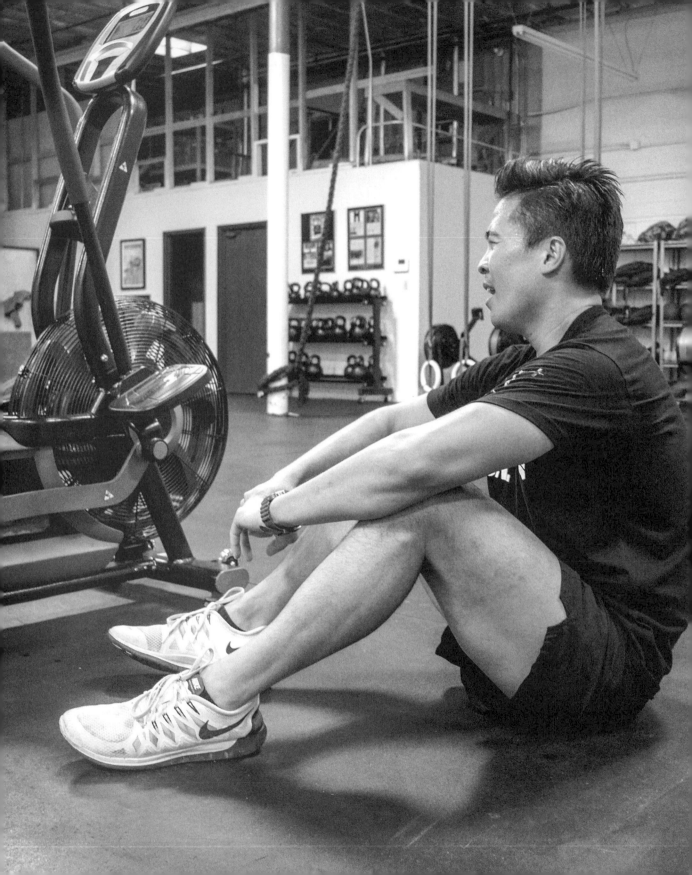

COOLDOWNS

A postworkout cooldown helps tune down your body after a workout and speeds your recovery, so you can improve quicker. Keep your cooldowns relaxed and simple—the hard work for the day is done.

When one of your workout days calls for a cooldown, you can choose from any of those below.

Cooldown 1
SHORT AND SWEET

DIRECTIONS

Walk or ride an exercise bike for 5 minutes.

1. Walk or Bicycle

Time: 5 Minutes

Cooldown 2
THE STANDARD

DIRECTIONS

Run on a treadmill, ride a bike, or row at a comfortable pace for 10 minutes.

1. Run, Bicycle, or Row

Time: 10 Minutes

Cooldown 3
FOR THE COMMITTED

DIRECTIONS

Run or row for 20 minutes, focusing on using perfect form.

1. Run or Row

Time: 20 Minutes

EXERCISES

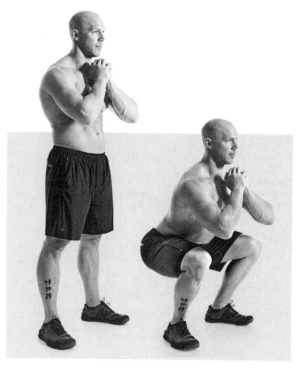

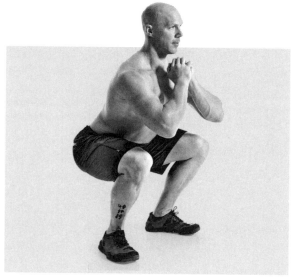

Air Squat

Stand with your feet slightly wider than shoulder-width apart, toes forward, and your hands clasped in front of you. Push your hips back and bend your knees as if you're about to sit in a chair, and lower your body. Keep your torso as upright as possible. Go as low as you can, pause, and then push back up to the starting position.

Air Squat Hold

Stand with your feet slightly wider than shoulder-width apart, toes forward, and your hands clasped in front of you. Push your hips back and bend your knees as if you're about to sit in a chair, and lower your body until your thighs are parallel to the floor or below your knees. Keep your torso as upright as possible. Hold the position.

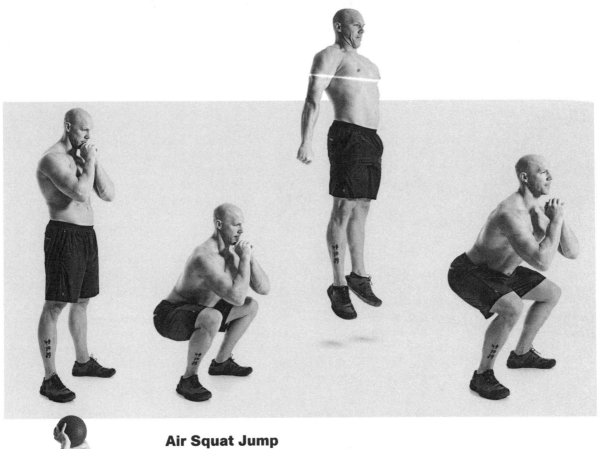

Air Squat Jump

Stand with your feet slightly wider than shoulder-width apart, toes forward, and your hands clasped in front of you. Push your hips back, dip your knees, and lower your body until your thighs are parallel with the floor or below your knees. Explosively jump as high as you can, your arms extending straight down toward the floor. Land softly, and repeat.

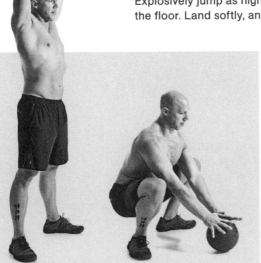

Ball Slam

Hold a medicine ball at waist level, and stand with your feet shoulder-width apart. While keeping your elbows slightly bent, explosively lift the ball overhead, and then slam it to the floor in front of you as hard as you can. Squat as you slam, dropping your hips toward the floor and grab the ball to repeat.

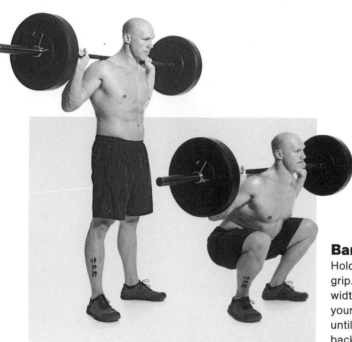

Barbell Back Squat

Hold a barbell across your back using an overhand grip. Your feet should be slightly wider than shoulder-width apart. Keep your head up and chest high, push your hips back, bend your knees, and lower your body until your thighs are at least parallel to the floor. Push back to the starting position.

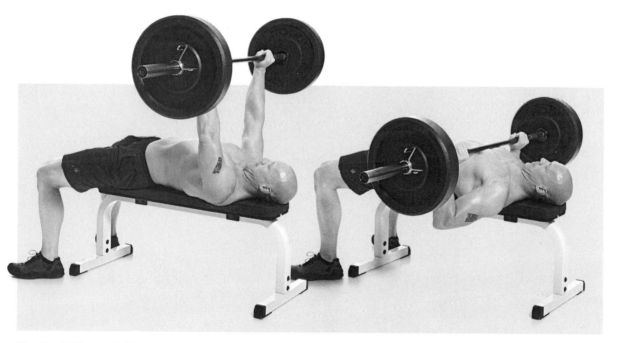

Barbell Bench Press

Lie with your back on a bench, holding a barbell overhead using an overhand grip that's just beyond shoulder-width apart. Lower the bar to your chest, and then push it back to the starting position.

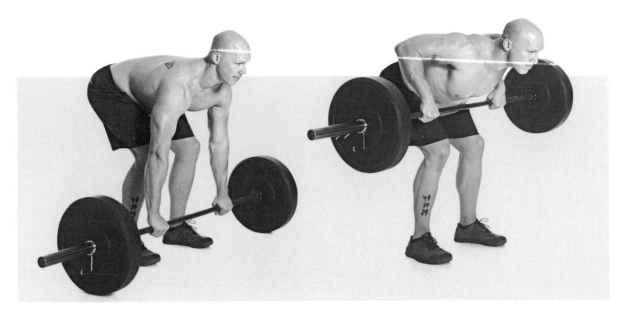

Barbell Bent Row

Grab a barbell with an overhand grip that's just beyond shoulder-width apart. Keeping your back naturally arched, bend at your hips and knees and lower your torso so it's almost parallel to the floor. Let the bar hang, slightly touching the floor, and then pull it toward your upper abs. Pause, and slowly lower the bar.

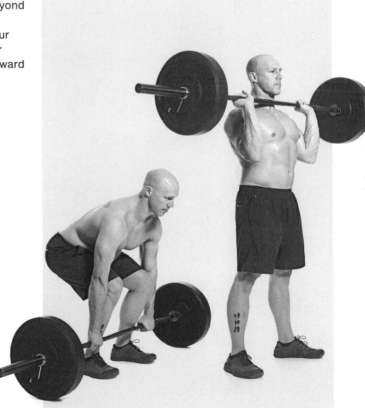

Barbell Clean

Place a loaded bar on the ground. Push your hips back, bend your knees, and grasp it with an overhand grip, at arm's length in front of you. Explosively push your hips forward and stand, pulling the bar up to shoulder height. "Catch" it up near your neck, your elbows under the bar.

Barbell Deadlift

Stand in front of a barbell, the bar touching your shins. Bend at your hips and knees and grab the bar overhand, your hands about shoulder-width apart. Keep your low back straight and brace your core as you pull your torso back and up, thrust your hips forward, and stand up with the bar. Carefully lower the bar back to the floor, keeping it close to your body.

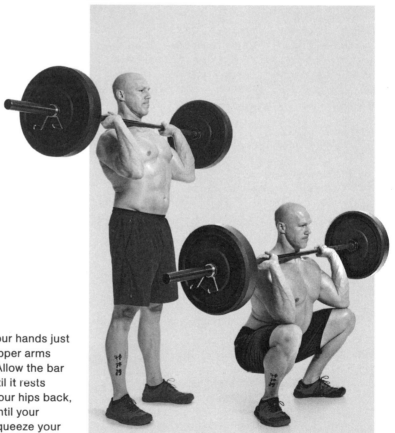

Barbell Front Squat

Hold a barbell using an overhand grip, your hands just outside your shoulders, and raise your upper arms until they're almost parallel to the floor. Allow the bar to roll back to the tips of your fingers until it rests securely on your front shoulders. Push your hips back, bend your knees, and lower your body until your thighs are at least parallel to the floor. Squeeze your glutes as you return to the starting position.

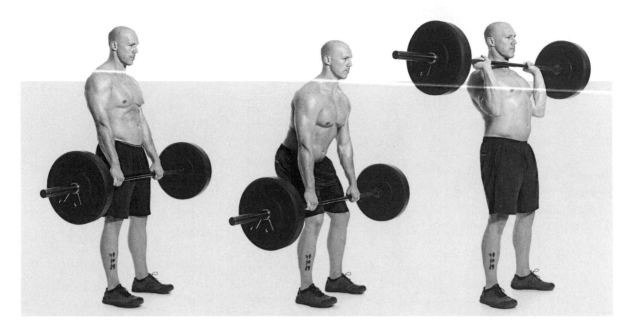

Barbell Hang Clean
Hold a barbell with an overhand grip, at arm's length in front of your hips. Push your hips back and slightly bend your knees. Now, explosively push your hips forward, pulling the bar up to shoulder height. "Catch" it up near your chest.

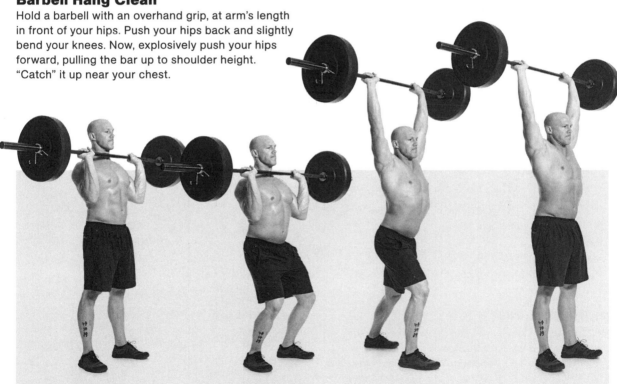

Barbell Jerk
Hold a barbell at shoulder height, your elbows bent and forearms vertical. Push your hips back as you explosively step your right foot forward and left foot back to generate momentum as you push the weight overhead.

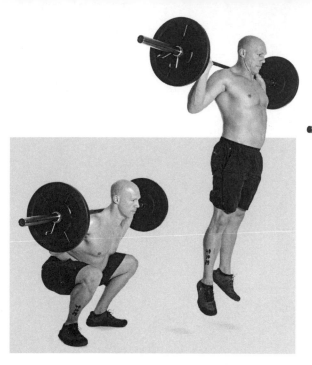

Barbell Jump Squat

Hold a barbell across your back, using an overhand grip. Your feet should be slightly wider than shoulder-width apart. Keep your head up and chest high, push your hips back, bend your knees, and lower your body until your thighs are about parallel with the floor. Explosively jump as high as you can. Softly land, squat, and jump again.

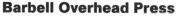
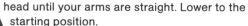

Barbell Overhead Press

Grab the barbell overhand with your hands just beyond shoulder-width apart, and hold it in front of your shoulders. Press the bar directly above your head until your arms are straight. Lower to the starting position.

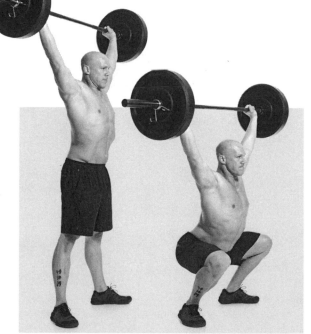

Barbell Overhead Squat

Hold a barbell over your head, using an overhand grip that's about twice shoulder-width. Your arms should be straight and your feet should be shoulder-width apart. Push your hips back and, while maintaining the natural arch in your lower back, squat as deeply as you can. Pause, and stand back up. Make sure that the bar doesn't move forward and that your arms remain perpendicular to the floor for the entire lift.

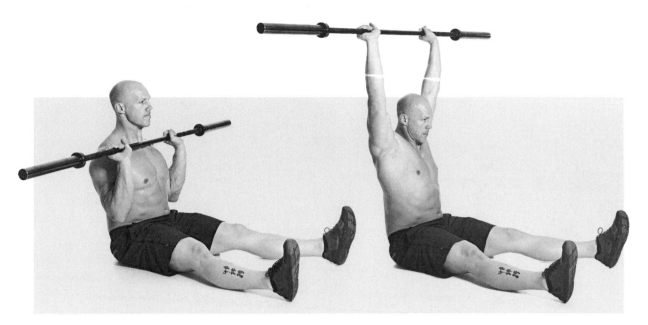

Barbell Z-Press

Sit on the floor with your legs straight out in front of you and your torso straight. Hold a barbell, using an overhand grip, at shoulder height, your elbows bent and forearms vertical. Press the bar overhead. Return to the starting position.

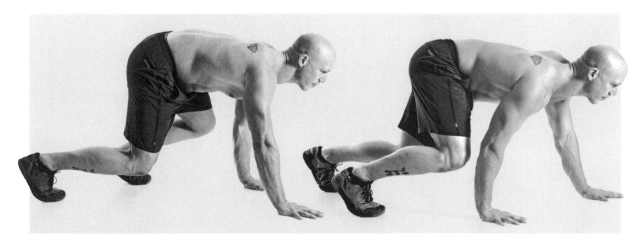

Bear Crawl

Assume a pushup position. Bring both your feet up so your knees and hips are bent 90 degrees. Move your right hand and left foot forward about 6 inches. Repeat with your left hand and right foot. Repeat the pattern in a "crawling" forward motion, keeping your back straight throughout.

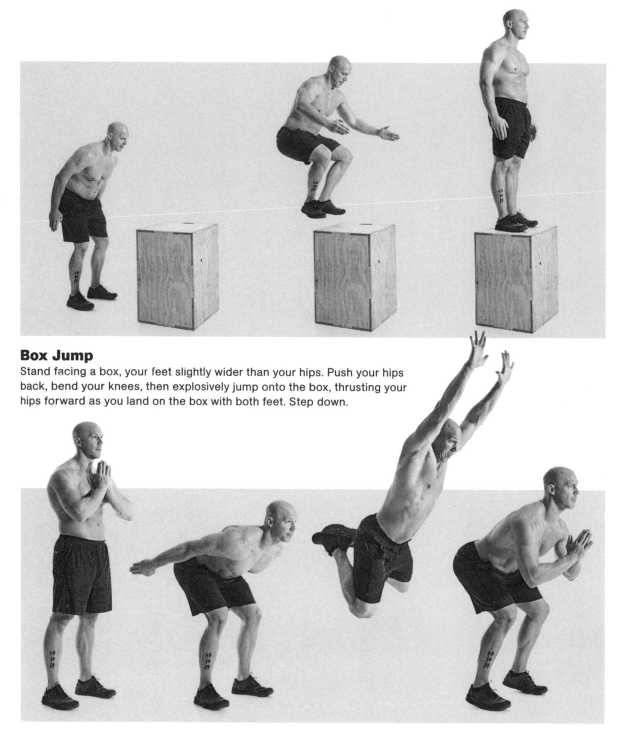

Box Jump

Stand facing a box, your feet slightly wider than your hips. Push your hips back, bend your knees, then explosively jump onto the box, thrusting your hips forward as you land on the box with both feet. Step down.

Broad Jump

Stand with your feet hip-width apart, your hands in front of you. Push your hips and arms back, bend your knees, and explosively jump as far forward as you can.

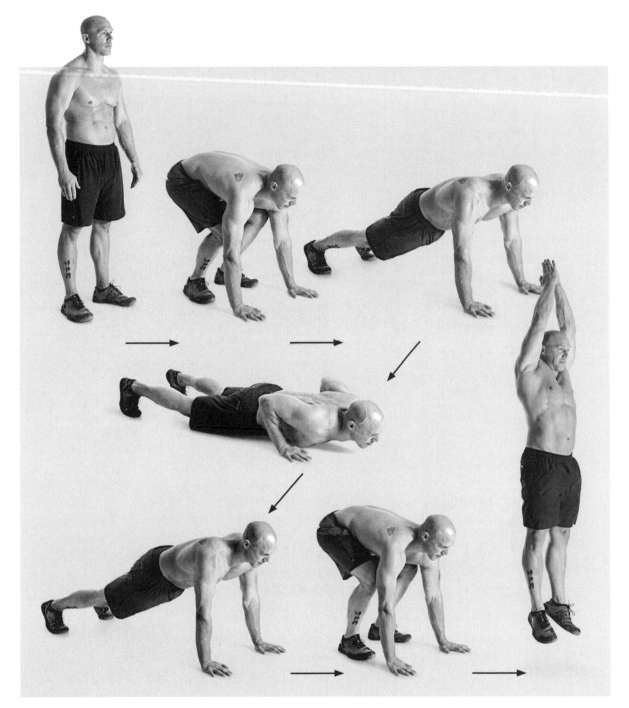

Burpee

Stand with your feet slightly beyond shoulder-width apart. Bend at your hips and knees, squat, and lower your body until you can place your hands on the floor. Kick your legs backward into a pushup position, and do a pushup. Immediately reverse the move and quickly stand up from the squat, then jump up at least 6 inches and clap your hands overhead.

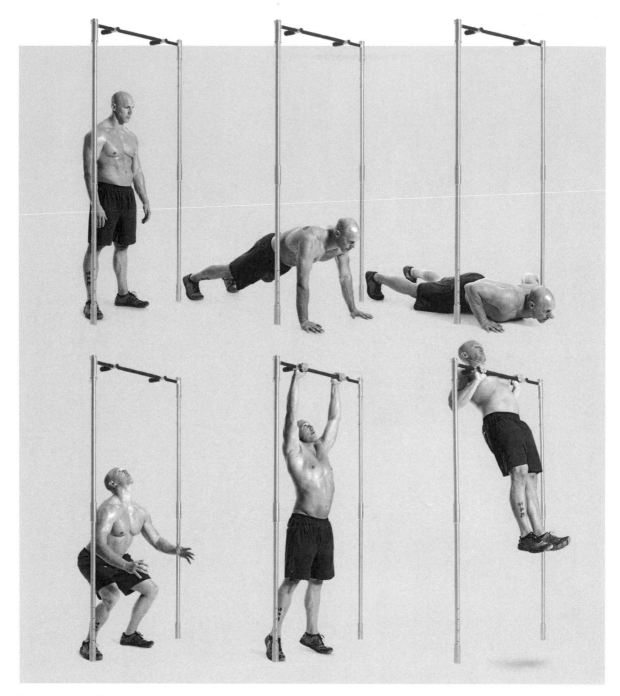

Burpee Pullup

Stand with your feet slightly beyond shoulder-width apart, a pullup bar above you. Bend at your hips and knees, squat, and lower your body until you can place your hands on the floor. Kick your legs backward into a pushup position, and do a pushup. Immediately reverse the move and quickly stand up from the squat, then jump up and grab the pullup bar. Pull your chest to the bar. Lower yourself, then drop back down to the ground.

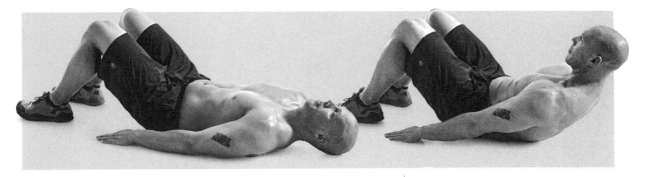

Curlup

Lie with your back and feet flat on the floor, your knees bent 90 degrees and your arms down by your sides. Curl your torso up, so your shoulders lift off the floor, keeping your head and neck straight. Pause, then lower yourself back down.

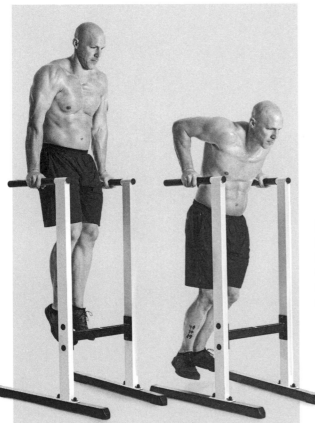

Dip

Grab the bars of a dip station and lift yourself so your arms are straight. Slightly flex your legs; this is the starting position. Shift your torso forward, bend your elbows, and lower yourself as far as you can without discomfort. Push back up to the starting position.

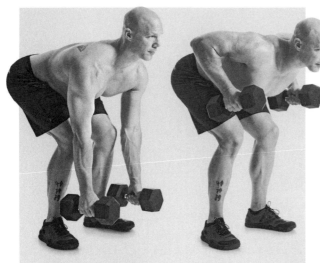

Dumbbell Bent Row

Holding a pair of dumbbells with your knees slightly bent, bend at your hips and lower your torso until it's almost parallel to the floor. This is the starting position. Bend your elbows and pull the dumbbells to the sides of your torso. Pause, and then slowly lower them.

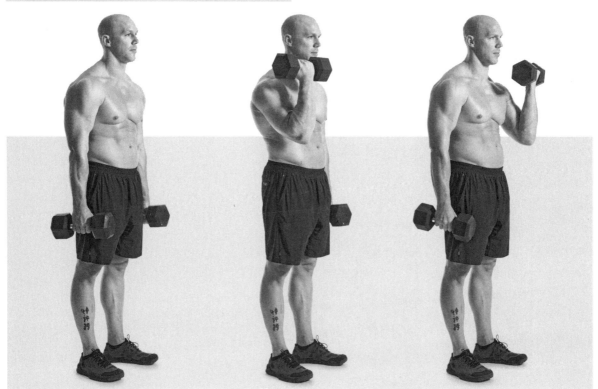

Dumbbell Biceps Curl

Grab a pair of dumbbells and let them hang next to your sides. Bend your right arm and curl the dumbbell as close to your shoulder as you can with your palms facing you. Pause, and slowly lower the weight back to the starting position. Repeat with your left arm.

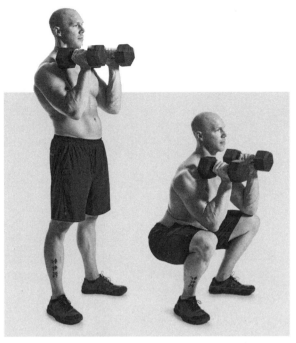

Dumbbell Front Squat

Hold a pair of dumbbells in front of you with your palms facing each other and one end of each dumbbell resting against the meatiest part of your shoulders. Push your hips back, bend your knees, and lower your body into a squat, without moving the dumbbells. Keep your torso as upright as possible. Go as low as you can without rounding your back, then push back up.

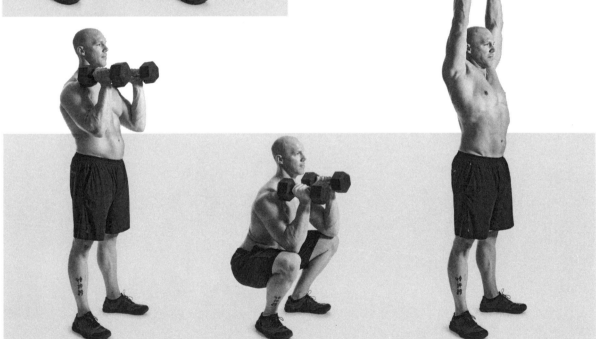

Dumbbell Front Squat Push Press

Hold a pair of dumbbells in front of you with your palms facing each other and one end of each dumbbell resting against the meatiest part of your shoulders. Push your hips back, bend your knees, and lower your body into a squat, without moving the dumbbells. Keep your torso as upright as possible. Go as low as you can without rounding your back. Push up explosively, using your lower-body power to help press the dumbbells overhead. Lower the dumbbells.

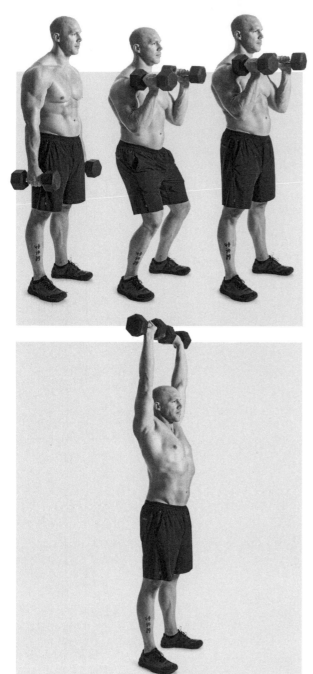

Dumbbell Hang Clean

Hold dumbbells with an overhand grip and at arm's length in front of your hips. Push your hips back, then explosively push them forward, pulling the dumbbells up to shoulder height. "Catch" them up near your shoulders, your palms facing each other.

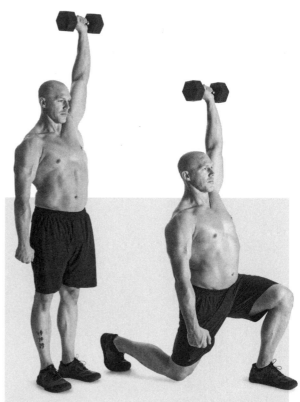

Dumbbell Overhead Hold

Grab two dumbbells, then press them overhead, with your palms facing forward. Hold the position, with your arms straight.

Dumbbell Overhead Lunge

Stand holding a dumbbell in your left hand with your arm straight over your head. Maintain that position as you take a large step forward with your left foot until your left front knee is bent 90 degrees and your right knee is an inch or two off the floor. Push back to the starting position, and repeat with the right leg.

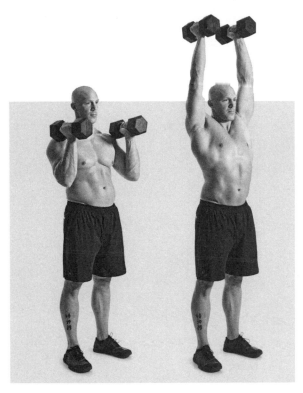

Dumbbell Overhead Press

Stand holding a pair of dumbbells just outside your shoulders, your arms bent, and your palms facing each other. Press the weights directly over your shoulders until your arms are straight. Slowly lower the dumbbells to the starting position.

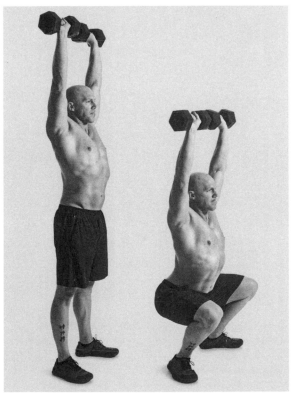

Dumbbell Overhead Squat

Hold dumbbells over your head, palms facing forward. Your arms should be straight and your feet shoulder-width apart. Push your hips back and, while maintaining the natural arch in your lower back, squat as deeply as you can. Pause, and stand back up. Make sure that your arms remain perpendicular to the floor for the entire lift.

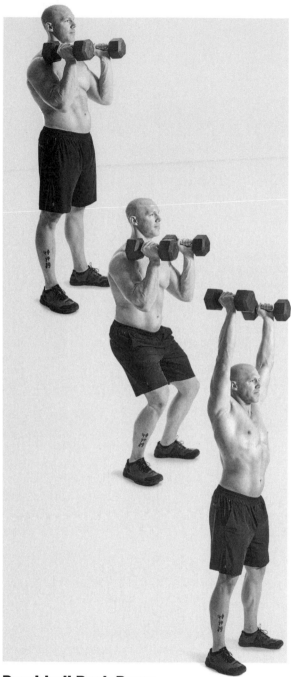

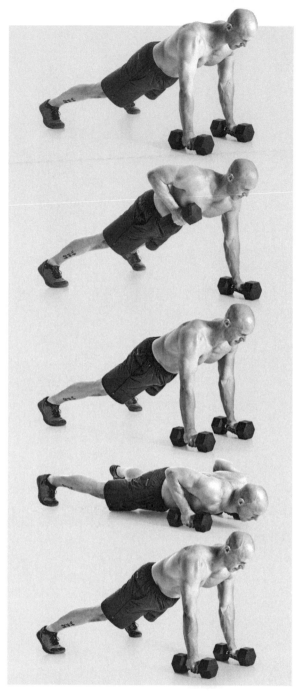

Dumbbell Push Press

Stand holding a pair of dumbbells just outside your shoulders, your palms facing each other. Dip your knees and push up explosively, using your lower-body power to help press the dumbbells overhead. Lower the weight to the original position.

Dumbbell One-Arm Row to Pushup

Assume a pushup position, gripping dumbbells in your hands on the floor. Pull the right dumbbell up to the right side of your chest. Pause. Lower it. Complete a row with the left. Do a pushup.

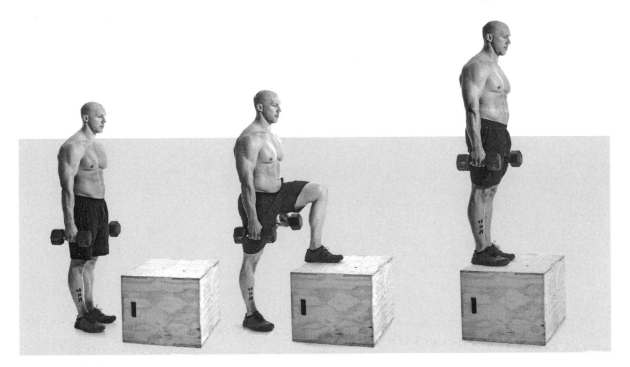

Dumbbell Stepup

Stand in front of a box or bench with your hands at your sides and your palms facing in. Hold a pair of dumbbells and place your left foot on a box or bench. Press through your left heel and step up, lifting yourself onto the box or bench, ending with both feet on the box or bench. Step off the box or bench and return to the starting position before switching legs.

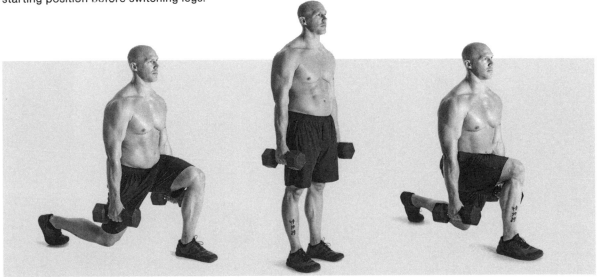

Dumbbell Walking Lunge

Stand holding a pair of dumbbells at your sides, palms facing in, and take a long step forward with your left foot, dropping your body until your left knee is bent about 90 degrees. Push up into a standing position, bringing your back foot forward. Repeat with your right foot. Alternate the leg you step forward with so that you're "walking" with each rep.

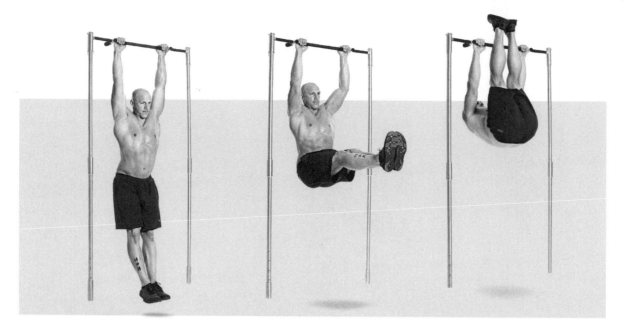

Feet-to-Hands

Hang from a pullup bar with an overhand, shoulder-width grip. Now raise your legs, bringing your feet to your hands. Pause, and lower your legs to the starting position.

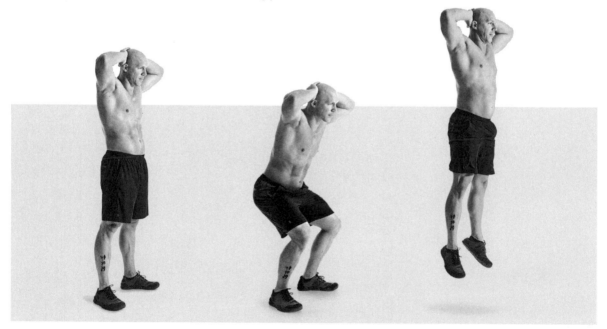

Frog Hop

Start in standing position with your hands behind your head and your torso straight. Lower yourself to half-squat position. If you have to slightly raise your heels from the floor to get into the position, that's okay. Then, explosively jump forward, landing back in the low squat position. You can also do this exercise jumping forward up a hill.

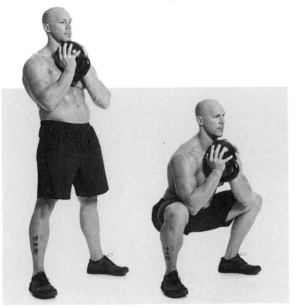

Goblet Squat

Grab a kettlebell or dumbbell and stand with your feet just beyond shoulder-width apart. Cup the weight with both hands and hold it vertically in front of your chest, your elbows pointing down. Keeping your back naturally arched, push your hips back, bend your knees, and lower your body until your knees are bent at least 90 degrees. Push yourself back to the starting position.

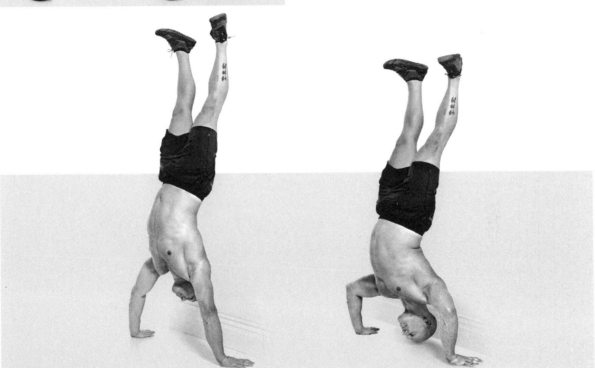

Handstand Pushup

Stand close to a wall, your back facing it. Put your hands on the ground, then place your feet on the wall. Walk your feet up the wall, so you're in a handstand position. With your feet resting on the wall and your arms straight, slowly bend your elbows and lower your head to the floor. Push back up, straightening your arms.

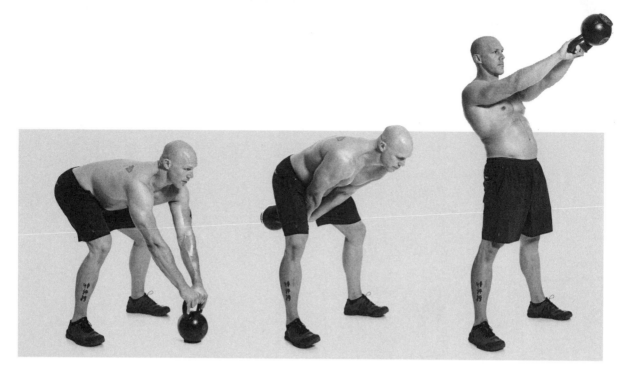

Kettlebell Swing

Start with a kettlebell on the ground in front of you, your hand clasping the handle, back straight, and knees bent. Without rounding your lower back, hike the kettlebell between your legs. Thrust your hips forward and let the weight swing to shoulder level as you stand up. Continue the movement, without letting the kettlebell touch the floor, swinging it like a pendulum.

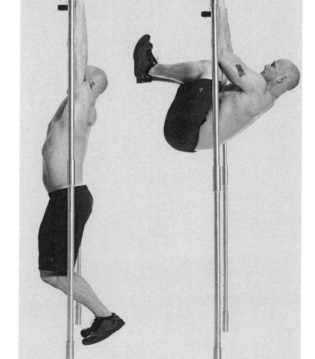

Knees-to-Elbows

Hang from a pullup bar, your body straight. Bring your knees up to your elbows, tucking your pelvis. Slowly lower your legs.

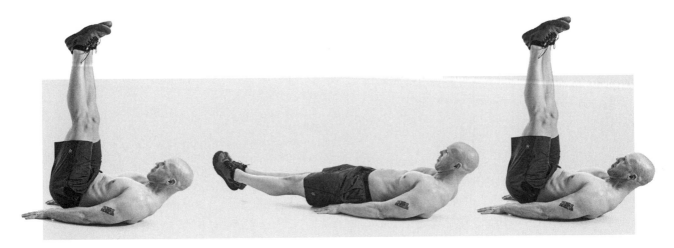

Leg Raise

Lie on your back, your hands at your sides and body straight. Raise your feet a few inches off the floor. This is the starting position. Keep your legs straight as you slowly raise them until they're vertical. Slowly reverse the movement and lower your legs back down.

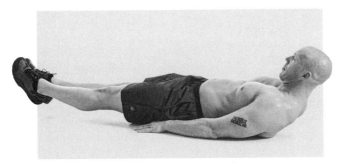

Leg Raise Hold

Lie on your back, your hands at your sides and body straight. Raise your feet a few inches off the floor while keeping your legs straight. Hold the position.

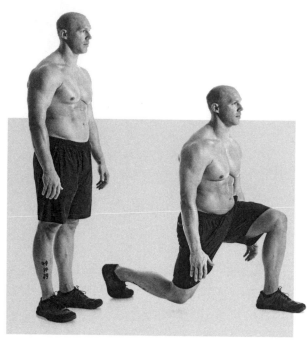

Lunge

Stand and take a large step forward. Your front thigh should be parallel to the floor and your back knee just off the floor. Return to a standing position. Repeat with your other leg.

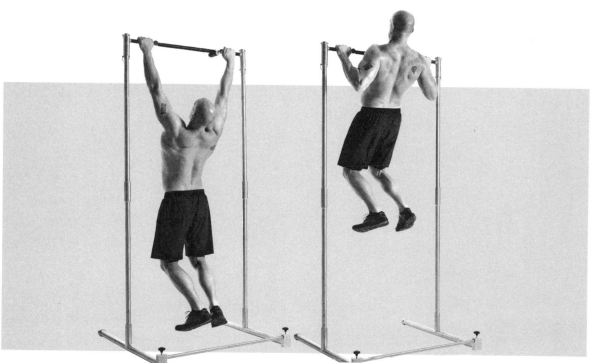

Pullup

Hang at arm's length from a pullup bar using an overhand grip with your hands slightly wider than shoulder-width apart. This is the starting position. Pull your chest to the bar as fast as you can, pause, and take a second to lower to the starting position.

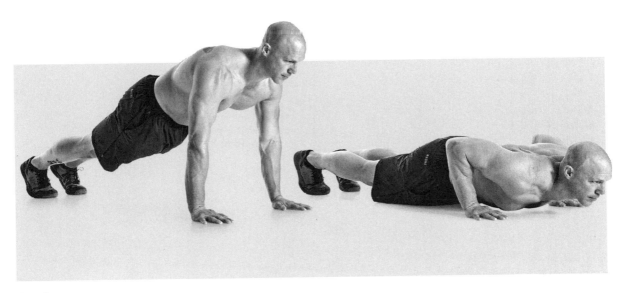

Pushup

Assume a pushup position, with your arms straight and hands below and slightly wider than your shoulders. Bend at the elbows and lower your body until your chest nearly touches the floor. Pause, and push your body back up.

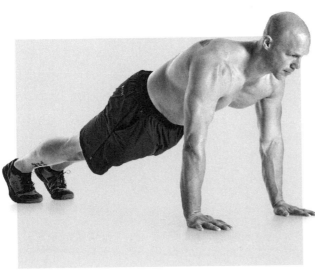

Pushup Position Plank

Assume a pushup position, your arms and torso completely straight. Hold the position.

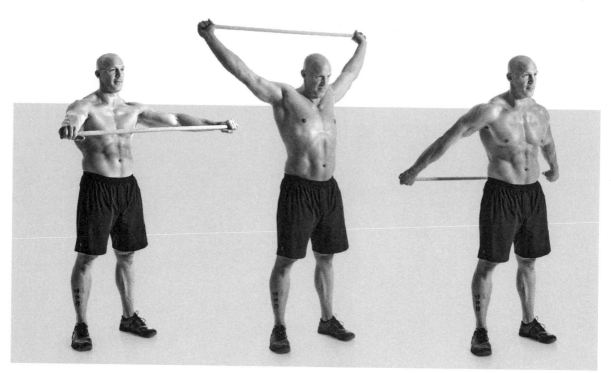

Shoulder Dislocate

Hold a pipe, dowel, or band in front of you with a wide overhand grip. Keep your arms straight throughout as you slowly arc the bar over and back behind your body, feeling the stretch in your shoulders. Slowly return to the starting position.

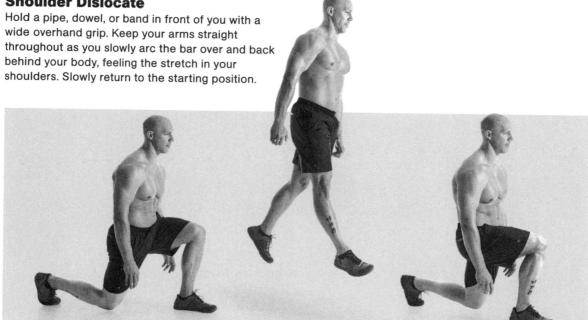

Split Jump

Step forward with your left foot and lower your body into a lunge, your front knee bent 90 degrees. Jump explosively, and switch leg positions in midair. Land in a lunge, with your right leg in front of your left. Repeat, alternating back and forth.

Stepup

Stand in front of a box or bench with your hands at your sides and your palms facing in. Place your left foot on the box or bench. Press through your left heel and step up, lifting yourself onto the box or bench, ending with both feet on the box or bench. Step off the box or bench and return to the starting position before switching legs.

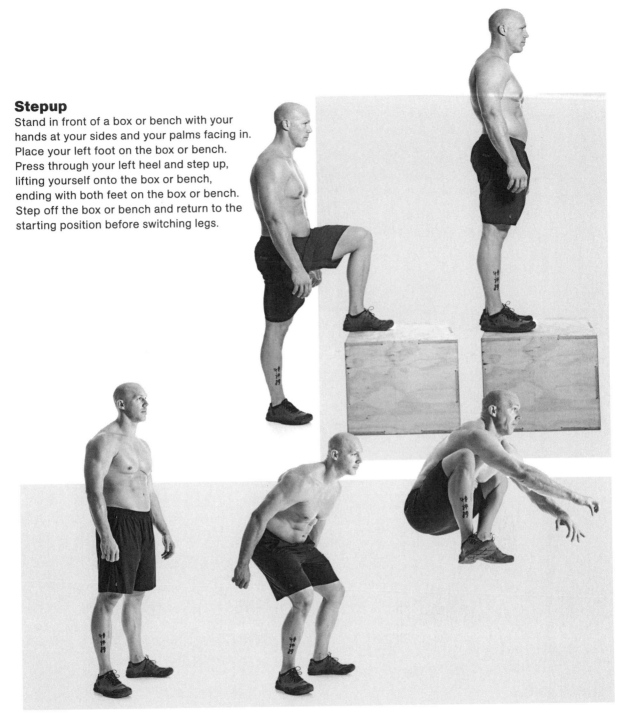

Tuck Jump

Stand with your feet shoulder-width apart. Take 2 small steps forward, then explosively jump as high as you can. As you rise, bring your knees up to your chest, "tucking" your pelvis. Extend your legs and return to the starting position.

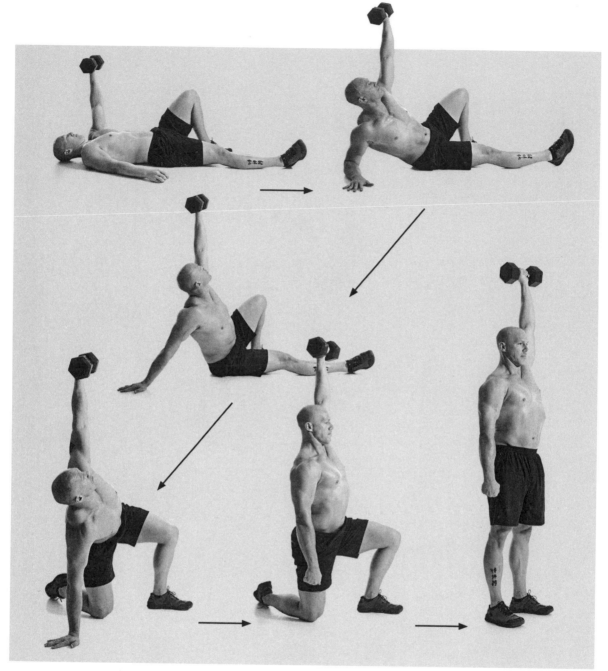

Turkish Getup

Lie on your back with your left leg bent and your right leg flat on the floor. Holding a dumbbell or kettlebell, raise your left arm straight overhead. Roll toward your right side and prop yourself up on your right elbow. Raise onto your right hand and slide your right leg behind your body. From this kneeling position, stand up while keeping the weight above you at all times. Once you're standing, step back with your left leg and perform the movement in reverse to return to the starting position. Repeat on your other side.

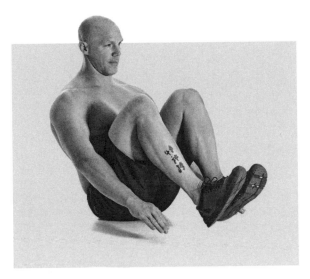

V-Sit Hold

Assume a V-sit position, your butt on the ground, knees to your chest, and feet just above the floor. Your arms should be at your sides, and hands just above the floor. Hold the position.

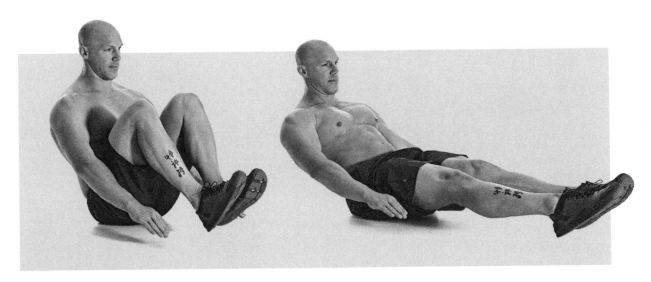

V-Sit Kickout

Assume a V-sit position, your butt on the ground, knees to your chest, and feet just above the floor. Your arms should be at your sides, and hands just above the floor. Slowly straighten your legs and lower your torso. Pause when your legs are straight, feet and upper back just a few inches above the floor. Reverse the move, pulling your knees back into your chest.

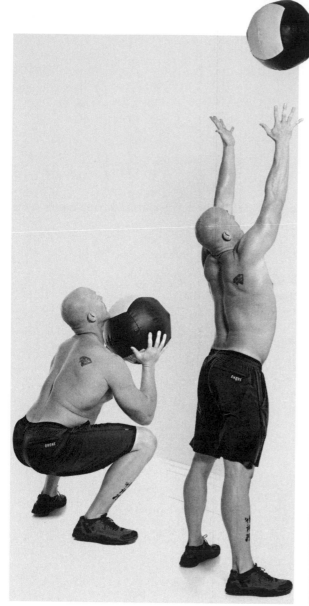

Wall Ball

Holding a medicine ball to your chest in front of a wall, bend your knees and push your hips back to squat down, then explosively push yourself back up. As you do, launch the ball as high as you can, slightly bouncing it off the wall so it falls back to you. Catch it and repeat.

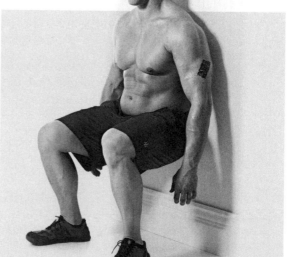

Wall Sit

Stand with your back to a wall. Push your hips back and lower your body until your thighs are parallel to the floor, your back resting against the wall. Hold the position.

ENDNOTES

SECTION I

1 V. K. Ranganathan. "From Mental Power to Muscle Power—Gaining Strength by Using the Mind," *Neuropsychologia* 42 (7), 2004: 944–56.

2 Sherry L Pagoto. "Twitter-Delivered Behavioral Weight-Loss Interventions: A Pilot Series," *JMIR Research Protocols* 4 (4), 2015 (Oct. 23): e123.

3 "Nutritional Supplements Flexing Muscles as Growth Industry," *Forbes*. Accessed 8/17/16. www.forbes.com/sites /davidlariviere/2013/04/18/nutritional-supplements-flexing-their-muscles-as-growth-industry/#1dd584c34255.

4 "Overweight and Obesity Statistics," NIH: National Institute of Diabetes and Digestive and Kidney Disorders. Accessed 8/17/16. www.niddk.nih.gov/health-information/health-statistics/Pages/overweight-obesity-statistics.aspx.

5 "108 Million Americans Now on a Diet, Highest Ever," PRWeb. Accessed 8/17/16. www.prweb.com/releases/2012/1 /prweb9112072.htm.

6 "NWCR Facts," The National Weight Control Registry. Accessed 8/20/16. www.nwcr.ws/research/.

SECTION II

1 James A. Levine. "What Are the Risks of Sitting Too Much?" Mayo Clinc. Accessed 11/2016. http://www.mayoclinic.org /healthy-lifestyle/adult-health/expert-answers/sitting/faq-20058005.

2 M. Chtara. "Effects of Intra-Session Concurrent Endurance and Strength Training Sequence on Aerobic Performance and Capacity," *British Journal of Sports Medicine* 39 (8), 2005 (Aug.): 555–60.

3 O. Storen. "Maximal Strength Training Improves Running Economy in Distance Runners," *Medicine and Science in Sports and Exercise* 40 (6), 2008 (June): 1087–92.

4 A. Sunde. "Maximal Strength Training Improves Cycling Economy in Competitive Cyclists," *Journal of Strength and Conditioning Research* 24 (8), 2010 (Aug.): 2157–65.

5 N. Bolandzadeh. "Resistance Training and White Matter Lesion Progression in Older Women: Exploratory Analysis of a 12-Month Randomized Control Trial," *Journal of the American Geriatric Society* 63 (10), 2015 (Oct.): 2052–60.

6 Eduardo B. Fontes. "Brain Activity and Perceived Exertion During Cycling Exercise: An fMRI Study." Accessed 11/2016. https://www.researchgate.net/publication/237013545_Brain_activity_and_perceived_exertion_during_cycling_exercise_An _fMRI_study.

SECTION III, PART I

1 Thomas M. Longland, Sara Y. Oikawa, Cameron J. Mitchell, Michaela C. Devries, and Stuart M. Phillips. "Higher Compared with Lower Dietary Protein during an Energy Deficit Combined with Intense Exercise Promotes Greater Lean Mass Gain and Fat Mass Loss: A Randomized Trial," *American Journal of Clinical Nutrition,* ajcn119339, first published online 1/27/16.

2 R. J. de Souza, A. Mente, A. Maroleanu, A. Cozma, V. Ha, T. Kishibe, E. Uleryk, P. Budylowski, H. Schunemann, J. Beyene, and S. S. Anand. "Intake of Saturated and Trans Unsaturated Fatty Acids and Risk of All Cause Mortality, Cardiovascular Disease, and Type 2 Diabetes: Systematic Review and Meta-Analysis of Observational Studies," *BMJ* 351, 2015 (Aug. 11): h3978.

3 D. Mozaffarian, M. B. Katan, A. Ascherio, M. J. Stampfer, and W. C. Willett. "Trans Fatty Acids and Cardiovascular Disease," *New England Journal of Medicine* 354 (15), 2006 (Apr. 13): 1601–13.

4 Angela K. Halyburton, G. D. Brinkworth, C. J. Wilson, M. Noakes, J. D. Buckley, J. B. Keogh, and P.M. Clifton. "Low and High-Carbohydrate Weight-Loss Diets Have Similar Effects on Mood but Not Cognitive Performance," *American Journal of Clinical Nutrition* 86 (3), 2007 (Sept.): 580–87.

5 Eric C. Westman, R. D. Feinman, J. C. Mavropoulos, M. C. Vernon, J. A. Wortman, W. S. Yancy, and S. D. Phinney. "Low-Carbohydrate Nutrition and Metabolism," *American Journal of Clinical Nutrition* 86 (2), 2007 (Aug.): 276–84.

6 F. Bellisle, R. McDevitt, A. M. Prentice. "Meal Frequency and Energy Balance" *British Journal of Nutrition*. 77 Suppl. (April 1997): S57–70. https://www.ncbi.nlm.nih.gov/pubmed/9155494. Accessed 11/2016.

7 Jim Giles. "Special Report Internet Encyclopaedias Go Head to Head," *Nature* 438, 2005 (15 Dec.): 900–901.

8 Malolan S. Rajagopalan, Vineet K. Khanna, Yaacov Leiter, Meghan Stott, Timothy N. Showalter, Adam P. Dicker, and Yaacov R. Lawrence. "Patient-Oriented Cancer Information on the Internet: A Comparison of Wikipedia and a Professionally Maintained Database," *Journal of Oncology Practice* 7 (5), 2011 (Sept.): 319–23.

SECTION III, PART 2

1 M. D. Milewski, D. L. Skaggs, G. A. Bishop, J. L. Pace, D. A. Ibrahim, T. A. Wren, A. Barzdukas. "Chronic Lack of Sleep Is Associated with Increased Sports Injuries in Adolescent Athletes," *Journal of Pediatric Orthopedics* 34 (2), 2014 (March): 129–33.

2 "Studies Link Fatigue and Sleep to MLB Performance and Career Longevity," *American Academy of Sleep Medicine*. Accessed 8/17/16. www.aasmnet.org/articles.aspx?id=3941.

3 Cheri D. Mah, MS; Kenneth E. Mah, MD, MS; Eric J. Kezirian, MD, MPH; and William C. Dement, MD, PhD. "The Effects of Sleep Extension on the Athletic Performance of Collegiate Basketball Players," *Sleep* 34 (7), 2011 (July 1): 943–50.

4 Thomas Reilly and N. Piercy. "The Effect of Partial Sleep Deprivation on Weight-Lifting Performance," *Ergonomics*, 37 (1), 1994 (Jan.): 107–15.

5 "Extra Sleep Improves Athletic Performance," *Science Daily*. Accessed 8/17/16. www.sciencedaily.com/releases/2008/06/080609071106.htm.

6 J. L. Broussard, D. A. Ehrmann, E. Van Cauter, E. Tasali, and M. J. Brady. "Impaired Insulin Signaling in Human Adipocytes after Experimental Sleep Restriction: A Randomized, Crossover Study," *Annals of Internal Medicine* 157 (8), 2012 (Oct. 16): 549–57.

7 "Blue Light Has a Dark Side," *Harvard Health Publications*, Harvard Medical School. Accessed 8/17/16. www.health.harvard.edu/staying-healthy/blue-light-has-a-dark-side.

8 J. B. Mann, K. R. Bryant, B. Johnstone, P. A. Ivey, and S. P. Sayers. "The Effect of Physical and Academic Stress on Illness and Injury in Division 1 College Football Players," *Journal of Strength and Conditioning Research* 30 (1), 2016 (Jan.): 20–25.

9 "Enhancing Low Back Health through Stabilization Exercises," University of Waterloo. Accessed 8/17/16. www.ahs.uwaterloo.ca/~mcgill/fitnessleadersguide.pdf.

10 G. Z. MacDonald, M. D. Penney, M. E. Mullaley, A. L. Cuconato, C. D. Drake, D. G. Behm, and D. C. Button. "An Acute Bout of Self-Myofascial Release Increases Range of Motion without a Subsequent Decrease in Muscle Activation or Force," *Journal of Strength and Conditioning Research* 27 (3), 2013 (March): 812–21.

11 Gregory E. P. Pearcey, MSc; David J. Bradbury-Squires, MSc; Jon-Erik Kawamoto, MSc; Eric J. Drinkwater, PhD; David G. Behm, PhD; and Duane C. Button, PhD. "Foam Rolling for Delayed-Onset Muscle Soreness and Recovery of Dynamic Performance Measures," *Journal of Athletic Training* 50 (1), 2015 (Jan.): 5–13.

SECTION IV

1 A. A. Crawley, R. A. Sherman, W. R. Crawley, and L. M. Cosio-Lima. "Physical Fitness of Police Academy Cadets: Baseline Characteristics and Changes during a 16-Week Academy," *Journal of Strength and Conditioning Research* 30 (5), 2016 (May): 1416–24.

ACKNOWLEDGMENTS

First and foremost I would like to thank my loving wife Lisa and my son Landon. Without the support of my family there is no way I could have completed this project. I would like to thank my mom and dad for always believing in me and molding me into the person I am today; Adam Campbell at Rodale Inc. for believing in my vision and commissioning this book; Michael Easter, my co-author, for the constant support, hard work, friendship, and not only guarding my vision but also for improving upon it; Jay Taylor and Shannon Baker from Lalo for offering their unconditional support in building the brand of Bobby Maximus; Matt Grossman for being a mentor and for some behind-the-scenes heavy lifting; Lisa Boshard, the founder of Gym Jones, for believing in me enough to place me in charge of the project. Finally, I'd like to thank everyone who has trained with me over the years and who has influenced me. I've been extremely fortunate to have had the opportunity to cross paths in a meaningful way with some of the best people in the world.

—Bobby Maximus

Thanks to Adam Campbell at Rodale Inc. for hiring me to work for *Men's Health* and taking a chance on me with this book; Bobby Maximus, for inviting me into his world and trusting me to portray it correctly; my mom, for her constant encouragement and for being the strongest person I know; and Leah, the dogs, and Nana for the support and laughs.

—Michael Easter

PHOTO CREDITS

INDEX

Boldface page references indicate photographs. <u>Underscored</u> references indicate boxed text.